Role of Parents in Adolescent Obesity

# 父母在青少年肥胖中的角色

温煦 著

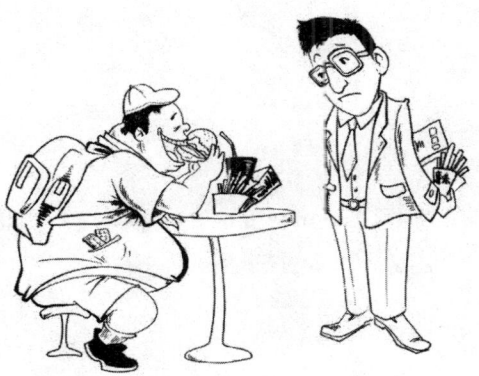

中央编译出版社
Central Compilation & Translation Press

# 写在前面的话

近年来，中国正面临青少年肥胖问题的严峻挑战。目前的研究显示，父母不仅可以在儿童肥胖控制方面发挥重要作用，还在儿童肥胖的发生和发展中扮演重要角色。首先，父母肥胖的遗传往往是引起儿童肥胖的重要因素之一。其次，父母为儿童提供或选择食物，这直接决定着儿童的能量摄入。此外，父母还充当子女的"榜样"和"权威"，他们的一举一动直接影响子女饮食和运动习惯的养成，他们的言行还影响着子女对于饮食和运动的态度和理念。然而，在中国，关于一些父母相关的因素与青少年体重水平之间的关系的研究报道还不够深入和全面。因此本研究的目的在于探讨中国父母对于孩子体重水平的认知、父母教养子女的行为、父母教养子女的方式与青少年肥胖的关系。为达到此研究目的，笔者进行了两项研究。

研究一（第三章）的目的在于验证父母教养子女的行为，父母对于孩子体重水平的认知以及父母教养子女的方式问卷的效度和信度。研究可分为以下几个步骤：第一，在前人研究的问卷中挑选一系列信度效度较好且适用于中国青少年和父母的问卷；第二，遵循跨文化翻译的基本步骤，将英文问卷翻译成中文；第三，邀请 5 名专家评估问卷的内容效度和问卷在中国人群中应用的可行性；第四，邀请 15 名青少年及其父母在试用问卷后进行简短访谈，考察问卷的可读性和文化相关问题，并根据他们的意见进行修改；第五，招募 127 对青少年（10 – 15岁）及其父母（赣州：62 对；汕头：65 对）进行问卷重测信度和内部一致性测试；第六，利用研究二的调查数据问卷的结构效度测试。10 个问卷题目因为内容效度不高或组内相关系数（ICC）低于 0.7 而被删除。亚量表的内部一致性均高于 0.6（范围：0.61 – 0.81），处于可以接受范围。结构效度测试中的模型拟合指数也显示问卷结构符合父母教养子女的行为和父母教养子女的方式的理论模型。因此本次研究的结果表明，这套问卷是可靠而有效的，可以应用于中国南方地区青少年及其父母。

研究二（第四、五、六章）旨在研究父母教养子女的行为、父母对于孩子体重水平的认知、父母教养子女的方式与青少年肥胖发展的关系。研究对象是中国赣州市和汕头市的 2143 名青少年和 1869 名他们的父母。青少年的身高和体重由培训过的测量员量度。青少年的饮食习惯、体力活动水平、父母教养子女的行为、父母教养子女的方式、父母对于孩子体重水平的认知以及其他信息通过研究一验证的问卷收集。结果显示，几种父母教养子女的行为，包括"强迫孩子吃东西"和"饮食和运动监控"，与青少年的 BMI – Z 分的相关系数不高但具有统计学意义（范围：– 0.23 至 .09，p < 0.01）。分层多变量回归的结果显

示，两种父母教养子女的行为（包括"强迫孩子吃东西"和"饮食和运动监控"）可以预测青少年的 BMI – Z 分。根据计算 Kappa 系数的结果，父母对于孩子体重水平的认知与青少年实际体重水平的一致性较差（Kappa = 0.221，p < 0.01）。而且，对于孩子体重水平的认知正确与错误的两类父母在父母教养子女的行为上有差异，且差异具有显著性。研究还发现，父母教养子女的方式可以调节青少年饮食习惯、身体活动水平、体重水平与父母教养子女的行为的关系。如，研究发现，当父母的关爱增强时，父母控制青少年不健康食品摄入的教养行为与青少年饮食习惯的正相关关系被加强了。本次研究的数据表明：父母教养子女的行为与青少年肥胖的发展相关微弱但具有统计学意义。许多父母对于孩子体重水平的认知不准确。父母教养子女的行为可能与父母对于孩子体重水平的认知有关。青少年的饮食习惯、体力活动水平以及部分父母教养子女的行为与父母教养子女的方式有关，但未发现父母教养子女的方式与青少年体重水平直接相关。

# 序　言

温煦博士毕业于香港中文大学，获得哲学博士，现为浙江大学讲师，在儿童肥胖研究领域有颇多建树，今以其学术研究心得著书造福国民，促进国民整体健康，值得肯定，本人亦深感荣幸能为本书作序。

近年，肥胖症（Obesity）成为了影响人类健康的严重问题之一，而且其影响是全球性的，因此"Globesity"成为了新兴的词汇，意思即"全球性肥胖症"（Global + Obesity）。2012年，世界卫生组织指出，自1980年到现在，全球肥胖人口增加了一倍，成为21世纪人类健康的公敌。据我国人民网于2011年的报道，肥胖人口近15年来以每年1.2%增长，使中国目前达到3.25亿肥胖人口，这数字在未来20年还会增加一倍。而我国儿童肥胖的增长速度，更是各年龄族群中之冠，值得担忧。肥胖症比起其他常见疾病例如心血管病和糖尿病或许更可怕，原因是许多人并没有意识到肥胖是一种疾病，误以为肥胖只是一种普通不过的现象，甚至以为肥胖是福。其实肥胖是现今大部分都市病的主凶，它能诱发多种心血管疾病，诸如心脏病、冠心病、高血压、糖尿病等多种疾病。肥胖症是一种慢性病，在日常生活中，不知不觉地慢慢累积而来，是经过多年来不健康的生活模式，习惯了吃得太多，活动得太少，于是把所吸收过多能量，转化成为身体脂肪储存，身体渐胖。长此以往，肥胖症到了难于逆转的地步。因此，要干预肥胖症，最好从儿时入手，如能在儿童时期控制了肥胖的问题，养成良好的生活习惯，长大了便更能保持健康的体型，远离肥胖问题。

那么，如何控制儿童肥胖，本书作者温煦博士有独特的见解。过去数十年的文献都会介绍各种控制儿童肥胖的干预手段，一般都是要肥胖儿童参与特别训练，限制他们的饮食，增加他们的体力劳动，于是肥胖儿童艰辛地熬过了地狱式的减肥课程，体重可能减少了。但是，当减肥特训一停止，儿童便再按捺不住已往的艰辛，放肆地大吃大喝，更惧怕了运动，于是肥胖问题反弹，甚至比之前更甚。其实儿童肥胖的主因往往并不是儿童自己造成的，而是他们生活的环境所致，尤其是他们的父母从小养育他们的方式。因此，温煦博士认为，要真正有效控制儿童肥胖，应从他们的父母入手。父母是控制儿童的饮食和安排儿童每天体能活动量的主要代理人。如父母懂得怎样从小给予子女正确的饮食和体能活动，并经常有意识地避免会导致儿童肥胖的不健康生活模式，那么其子女便能在最自然的健康生活模式下成长，于是肥胖的情况便能及早在不知不觉间得到控制，那么一来，儿童便不再需要面对那些枯燥无味、非人生活的减肥课程了。

盼望这本书能为家长们带来有用的理论和实践建议，使你们的子女能健康地成长，让中国未来新一代更健康。

许世全　教授
香港中文大学　体育运动科学系　教授
美国运动医学学院　院士
2012 年 6 月 26 日

# 目　录

# 表索引

# 第一章　前　言

## 第一节　研究的背景

在过去的几十年中，青少年肥胖问题已经成为世界范围内的公共卫生问题。有研究预测，在全世界有 1/10 的学龄儿童超重（Lobstein, et al., 2004）。在香港，青少年肥胖的流行趋势从 1994 年到 2007 年已经增长到了 70%（Yeung & Hui, 2007）。自 1989 年到 1997 年，中国城镇地区的肥胖流行率从 1.5% 增加到了 12.6%，超重的患病率从 14.6% 增加到了 28.6%（Luo & Hu, 2002）。

由于肥胖发病率的继续增长，儿童肥胖增加了成人肥胖和许多相关疾病的风险（Choudhary, et al., 2007; Gunnell, et al., 1998），数以千计的研究致力于找出引起儿童肥胖的原因和合适的治疗方法。在这些研究中，有两个有趣的现象被发现：第一，父母身材臃肿的孩子看起来有更高的发展成肥胖的风险（Treuth, et al., 2003）；第二，父母是否参与到干预中和孩子的减肥效果有关（McLean, et al., 2003）。这些研究表明，父母可能在青少年肥胖的病因和预防中扮演着重要的角色。

　　肥胖是由多种原因引起的长期能量摄入过剩造成的（Barlow & the Expert Committee，2007）。引起青少年儿童肥胖的几种可能的危险因素已经被发现，包括缺乏身体锻炼（Rennie，et al.，2005），长时间观看电视（Danner，2008），大量摄入快餐（Bowman，et al.，2004），等等。显然，家长可能与这些因素中的大部分有关，具有潜在的调解或缓冲其中许多因素的影响的能力。研究发现，父母不仅在青少年儿童生活习惯的养成中扮演关键的角色，对青少年儿童的食物喜好和饮食习惯的发展也有影响（Rhee，2008）。此外，还发现父母喂养子女的行为（Faith，Berkowitz，et al.，2004）和父母自己的食物摄入量（Fisher，et al.，2002）可以影响青少年儿童的食物摄入量。另外，父母的支持（Prochaska，et al.，2002）和父母自己的身体活动（Yang，et al.，1996）也和青少年儿童的体重状况相关。这些研究提示，父母可以通过自己的行为来影响青少年儿童的体重状况。

　　由于父母教养子女的行为在决定青少年儿童肥胖方面也发挥着重大作用，第一个问题就是什么可以激发父母去选择和调整他们的行为。父母积极乐意地去调整他们的行为可能是预防青少年肥胖的重要的过程之一。近来的研究表明，父母对子女体重的认知和父母是否乐意帮助他们的子女减肥具有相关性（Rhee，et al.，2005）。遗憾的是，近来的研究指出大多数的父母对子女的体重认识存在误解（Eckstein，et al.，2006；Etelson，et al.，2003；Ward，2008）。但是，父母对子女的体重认识存在误解是否会影响他们教养子女的行为？是否又会影响子女肥胖的发展？目前的研究还没有很好地回答这些问题。

父母教养子女的行为是父母做了什么，而父母教养子女的方式则是父母怎么做的。父母教养子女的方式提供了父母的行为是如何表达及儿童如何理解的情感背景（Rhee，2008）。研究还发现父母教养子女的方式和儿童肥胖有相关性。例如，有研究发现，在控制了儿童时期的年龄、性别、体重指数（BMI）和社会背景等因素后，父母对子女的放任会导致青少年肥胖的发生风险升高（Lissau & Sørensen，1994）。还有学者发现，与民主型母亲抚养的儿童相比较，专制型母亲抚养长大的儿童有更高的体重超重风险（Rhee，Lumeng，Appugliese，Kaciroti，& Bradley，2006）。因此，包括了针对父母教养子女的行为和方式干预方案要比单独针对父母教养子女的行为的干预方案更为有效（Rhee，et al.，2006）。

父母教养子女的行为和方式受到不同文化的影响。在中国，传统的中国教育受儒家思想的影响超过 2000 年。在传统的中国家庭里，父母和子女之间关系紧密，而且父母直接主导着他们子女的生活方式。即使在今天，虽然中国社会已经深受西方的影响，但是许多中国父母的理念和行为仍然深受传统儒家思想的影响（Holroyd，2003；P. Wu，et al.，2002；Xu，et al.，2005）。中国父母教养子女的方式特点是"严格的"、"高控制的"和"专制的"（Lin & Fu，1990；Steinberg，et al.，1992）。研究指出，美国人重视培育孩子自身的天赋，中国人则更重视自律和顺从父母，这也是中国文化的重要组成部分（Chao，1994；F. M. Chen & Luster，2002）。不过，在中国只有少部分学者调查了父母教养子女的行为和方式与青少年肥胖之间的相关性。例如，一项基于163个中国孩子和他们在台湾地区和美国的母亲的研究表明，父母教养子女方式的民主程度与儿童体重水平存在相关性（J. L. Chen & Kennedy，2004）。另一名香港学者则发现，父母可能会影响超重青少年对身体活动的兴趣（Lau，et al.，2007）。

尽管中国的一些学者已经研究了父母教养子女的行为和对儿童肥胖状况的影响，但仍有许多问题没有很好地回答。比如，在过去的30年，随着中国大陆在20世纪70年代开始实施计划生育政策，这导致了中国的人口自然增长率急剧下降（Jing，1994），同时也影响了数百万中国父母教养子女的行为和方式。如今，许多中国孩子在家中被父母视为小皇帝和小公主。这和传统的中国父母的教养子女方式显著不同。此外，数百年来，中国的父亲和母亲所扮演的角色也是有所不同的（Berndt，et al.，1993），这也提示，在中国，父亲和母亲在教养子女的行为和方式上可能是不同的。但是，我们并不知道父母在教养子女的行为和方式上的差异是否与儿童肥胖的发展存在联系。因此，仍然需要深入研究中国父母教养子女的行为、父母教养子女的方式、父母对孩子体重的认知与青少年的体重水平之间的关系。

此外，虽然已经有了一些成熟的问卷和量表可以衡量父母教养子女的行为和方式（Birch，et al.，2001；Golan & Weizman，

1998；Hughes, et al. , 2003），但是大部分关于父母教养子女行为和儿童肥胖的研究仅仅关注了一个方面，即家长的控制（Hughes, et al. , 2008）。例如，儿童饮食调查问卷（CFQ）是一种常常用于测量父母的喂养子女的理念、态度和行为的工具。然而，验证性因子分析的结果显示，儿童饮食调查问卷七个维度中的四个都集中在父母的控制措施上（Birch, et al. , 2001）。另外，考虑到文化背景的不同，没有进行没有有效性和可靠性测试之前，在西方国家应用成熟的问卷调查也不能直接应用于中国人群的测试。

综上所述，现在仍有几个研究问题尚未解决。首先，目前还没有可以用于测量中国父母教养子女的行为、父母教养子女的方式、父母对孩子体重水平认知的问卷。第二，父母教养子女的行为、父母教养子女的方式、父母对孩子体重水平认知与儿童的体重状况之间的关系仍不清楚。第三，国外针对父母教养子女行为和方式的报道较多，但是对于中国父母的教养子女的行为、教养子女的方式以及父母对子女体重水平的认知的研究报道仍然非常少。因此，在本次研究中，提出了几个研究问题。第一，中国父母教养子女的行为和青少年肥胖的发展是否存在相关？第二，中国父母错误判断子女体重状况的情况是否普遍？父母对子女体重的认知是否和父母教养子女的行为存在相关？第三，父母教养子女的方式是否和青少年肥胖相关？不同教养子女方式的父母在教养子女的行为上是否存在差异？

# 第二节　研究目的

鉴于目前关于中国父母对子女体重水平的认知、父母教养子女的行为、教养子女的方式和青少年的体重水平的相关研究还比较少，测量问卷比较缺乏的现状，因此，本研究的主要目的是：1. 检验用于测量中国父母教养子女的行为、父母教养子女的方式、父母对孩子体重水平认知的调查问卷的有效性和可靠性；2. 确定中国父母教养子女的行为、父母教养子女的方式、父母对孩子体重水平认知与青少年的体重状况之间的关系。

# 第三节　研究意义

本研究主要有以下意义：1. 本研究所验证的调查问卷将成为对未来研究人员进行相关研究和评估的重要工具。2. 帮助父母选取有效的教养子女的行为和方式，以防治子女的肥胖问题。3. 为青少年肥胖的控制和干预策略的制订提供重要信息。4. 为国家健康政策的制订提供有益的参考。

# 第四节　研究假设

**设置的原假设：**

1. 对于青少年和父母的调查问卷的重测信度、内部的一致性和结构效度不理想。

2. 父母对他们子女体重状况的认知和青少年实际体重状况不一致。

3. 父母教养子女的行为和青少年体重状况之间不存在相关性。

4. 父母教养子女的方式和青少年体重状况之间不存在相关性。

# 第五节　操作定义

## 一、父母对青少年体重状况的认知

在本次研究中，父母对子女的认知被定义为父母对他们子女体重水平的认识和分类的自我报告（Warschburger & Kroller, 2009）。

## 二、父母教养子女的行为

在本次研究中，父母教养子女的行为的定义是：可能会影响孩子的体重状况的父母的行为或反应，包括家长对孩子的饮食策略，以及对孩子的体育活动以及少动久坐行为的反应（Rhee, 2008）。

## 三、父母教养子女的方式

在本次研究中，父母教养子女的方式被定义为孩子报告的父母教养子女的模式，该模式包含父母表达他们教养子女行为时带有的情感，以及被青少年理解到的态度（Darling & Steinberg，1993）。

## 四、青少年肥胖

在这项研究中，青少年肥胖被定义为体重指数（BMI）高于相应年龄和性别组别的学龄儿童和青少年的国际成长标准中的临界值（Butte，et al.，2007；De Onis，et al.，2007）。

# 第六节　研究的不足

首先，由于本研究是一项确定中国的青少年肥胖和父母教养子女的行为。父母教养子女的方式之间关系的横断面研究，不能提供变量之间因果关系的信息。其次，当前学者收集的大部分数据都是基于参与者的主观报告。然而，有时自我报告的主观数据可能反映了参与者自己理想化的数据，而不是实际的现实。有时，参与者更愿意给的答复是社会可接受的，而不是真实的情况。

# 第七节　研究的局限

首先，由于中国国土辽阔，而且中国城市青少年肥胖的发病率高于农村地区，本研究仅仅选取中国南部的两个城市参与该研究。此外，本研究仅招募了初中一年级和二年级的学生作为研究对象。因此，该研究的结果不一定适用其他地区其他年龄段的青少年和父母。

其次，本研究采用了体重指数（BMI）而不是体脂百分比作为衡量青少年和他们父母身体肥胖程度的指标。因为 BMI 并不是身体成分的直接指标，所以有时候，体重指数（BMI）较高并不等同于机体脂肪含量高。

第三，被招募来进行调查问卷的可靠性测试的青少年及其父母，被介绍参加这项研究时，并不知道需要在两周的间隔时间重复完成一份调查问卷。

# 第二章　文献综述

## 第一节　前　言

由于儿童肥胖可能导致成年肥胖，并且可能增加成年后患慢性疾病的风险，因此为了更好地控制成年人群中的肥胖率，目前急需采取儿童肥胖干预项目进行控制（Magarey, et al., 2003；Must & Strauss, 1999）。但是，许多干预项目都呈现出病人缺席、高退出率以及体重控制失败等特点（Stewart, et al., 2008）。因此，目前急需一些新型的、能够长期性执行并能够让受干预者持续参与的肥胖干预项目。

专家委员会对于儿童期肥胖的建议指出了父母参与在干预中的重要性（Barlow & the Expert Committee, 2007）。有些专家建议这种针对儿童期肥胖的项目应该以家庭为基础，至少有一位父母的参与，不然可能会导致干预失败（Dietz & Robinson, 2005；Robinson, 1999）。因此，基于家庭的干预，或甚至专门针对父母的干预项目可能是较为理想的长期儿童肥胖的干预项目。强有力的研究证据之一是来自 Epstein 等人的研究，该研究证明了一项长达 10 年的父母—孩子干预项目的有效性（Epstein, et al., 1990）。父母不仅在儿童期肥胖的治疗中扮演了关键性角色，而且在儿童期肥胖的起因和发展中也同样起着关键作用。父母自身的肥胖是影响子女体重水平，尤其是幼年子女体重的重要因素，并且这种影响会持续到子女成年。（Whitaker, et al., 1997）。父母为孩子提供食物或者替孩子选择食物。此外，父母可以起到行为榜样和权威人物的作用，不仅帮助孩子形成饮食和运动的习惯，而且还会影响孩子对饮食习惯和运动参与的态度与理念（Rhee, 2008）。

一些文献综述强调了父母观念、父母行为、教育方式以及其他一些与父母有关的因素和儿童期肥胖之间的联系（Faith, Scanlon, et al., 2004；Howard, 2007；Lindsay, et al., 2006；Rhee, 2008）。但是，虽然父母的影响对于儿童期肥胖是多方面的，大多数的研究综述仅仅研究了一个或两个因素。此外，很少有研究关注中国儿童和父母。因此，为了更好地理解父母肥胖与儿童期肥胖之间的关系，这篇综述致力于总结近些年关于儿童期肥胖和父母有关因素之间的关系，这些因素包括遗传、父母对于孩子体重的认知、父母对于营养和肥胖的观念和知识、父母教养子女的行为、父母教育子女的方式、家庭环境和一些其他相关因素。

# 第二节　遗传和儿童肥胖

在过去几年旦，儿童肥胖率的迅速增加经常被认为与环境的变化有关（Franzini, et al., 2009; Strauss & Knight, 1999）。但是，不是所有儿童都同样程度地受到不健康生活方式的影响。有一些儿童即使是在非常容易肥胖的环境中仍保持清瘦。对于这些孩子如何保持理想体重通常只有两种基础性解释（O'Rahilly & Farooqi, 2008）。首先，这些儿童的父母在子女的饮食和运动上总能一直做出正确的决定。另一个原因就是遗传。这些瘦的孩子可能在生物学上就与其他孩子不同，这种生物学差异通过某种机制使他们能够控制好体重问题。

## 一、遗传对儿童期肥胖的影响

### （一）基于父母—子女的研究

一项最近的基于 4884 名儿童的数据显示，母亲超重会影响所有儿童 BMI 指数的分布变化，而引起体重水平最高那部分儿童的 BMI 指数的增加幅度会更大（Toschke, et al., 2008）。但是，该研究同时也发现，"多吃少餐"、非母乳喂养、母亲怀孕期间吸烟、父母教育水平、长时间看电视等因素仅会导致体重水平最高那部分儿童的 BMI 指数的增加，而不是对所有儿童都有影响。一项纵向跟踪研究则发现，父亲的全身脂肪总量和体脂百分比可以影响他们女儿长期的全身脂肪总量和体脂百分比的变化（Figueroa-Colon, et al., 2000）。此外，另一项研究也显示，父母的标准化后的体重变化与子女出生后到 6 个月（$P < 0.001$）以及出生后到 24 个月（$P < 0.009$）的标准化后的体重变化均存在相关（Wrotniak, et al., 2004）。这一研究也显示父母和子女的体重之间是存在联系的。因而假如父母在基于家庭

的干预项目中成功减体重，那么子女也有可能从中获益。

类似的研究结果在中国也有报道。一项基于9325名6 – 8 岁儿童的横向研究显示，正常体重父母的子女儿童肥胖的发病率为 11.1％。但父母肥胖的子女儿童肥胖的发病率就高达 33.6%（Y. Yu，et al.，2002）。2002 年中国国家营养与健康调查的数据显示，当父母的体重越重，孩子体重超重的风险就越高（Y. Li，et al.，2007）。另一项对象为 11545 名 0 – 6 岁深圳儿童的调查则显示，有 13 个因素与儿童期肥胖有关，包括了父母超重，父亲受教育水平低，出生体重大于等于 4 公斤以及其他的一些因素（B. Chen，et al.，2008）。这些大样本的调查成功证明了在中国人群中儿童期肥胖与父母体重之间的显著相关。

有研究发现，孕期女性的脂肪增加，可能改变子宫内环境，增加子女发生肥胖的风险，使下一代的肥胖问题更趋严重（Levin，2000）。如果这种作用机制正确的话，那么母亲 BMI 与子女 BMI 的相关系数应高于父亲 BMI 与子女 BMI 的相关系数。但是，通过对 4654 户家庭的调查发现母亲—子女 BMI 和父母—子女 BMI 系数相比并没有明显的区别（Smith，et al.，2007）。因此，子女体重是否会被母亲怀孕时子宫内环境所影响还有待于进一步研究。

（二）基于双胞胎的研究

经典的基于双胞胎的研究是判断家庭成员间某种特质存在相关是基于遗传因素影响还是共同的环境因素影响的最有效的分析方法。与基于父母—子女模式的研究相比，双胞胎研究模式提供了一种独有的方式可以区别先天和后天因素影响。这种方法是以同卵双胞胎拥有相同的基因而异卵双胞胎只有一半相同基因为理论基础的（如果是基于遗传原因，则同卵双胞胎之间的相关应大于异卵双胞胎间的相关。而如果是环境原因，则同卵双胞胎之间的相关和异卵双胞胎间的相关之间的差异应不存在显著性。）（Hopper, et al., 2005）。通过超过25000对双胞胎和50000个生父母或养父母的研究，汇总下来同卵双胞胎加权后的相关系数为0.74，异卵双胞胎为0.32，兄弟姐妹为0.25，父母子女为0.19，收养关系为0.06，夫妻关系则为0.12（Maes, et al., 1997）。另一项研究通过DXA（双能X光吸收法）测量了双胞胎的全身脂肪和局部脂肪分布（Malis, et al., 2005）。研究结果同样显示，同卵双胞胎全身脂肪百分数的组内相关要高于以卵双胞胎全身脂肪百分比的组内相关。这些研究表明基因因素对身体脂肪的变化起着重要作用。

因为身体脂肪的百分比可以由遗传来解释，大多数的研究得出了相似的结论，那就是成年人体重的55%－86%是由遗传决定的（Fabsitz, et al., 1994；Faith, et al., 1999）。比如，有研究利用双胞胎模型用来判断遗传对于肥胖的影响，结果发现遗传系数为0.86（95%置信区间为0.77－0.94）（Bulik, et al., 2003）。近期一项对英国五千多对双胞胎的BMI和腰围的研究则发现，BMI和腰围由遗传决定的比例均为77%（Wardle, et al., 2008）。这些研究都证明了，遗传在肥胖的发展过程中起着非常重要的作用。

（三）研究的不足

基于父母—子女或双胞胎的研究中可能存在的其中一个不

足是父母—子女和兄弟姐妹之间的相关性完全无法区分遗传和环境的影响。在基于父母—子女或双胞胎的研究中，遗传性可能被高估，因为家庭成员之间不仅共享了相同的基因还分享了相同的环境。解决这个问题的办法之一是以存在收养关系的家庭作为研究对象。这种研究设计的方法背后的逻辑是孩子与生父母之间的相似性可以由共享基因来解释，而被收养的孩子与养父母之间的相似性可以由共享环境因素来解释。比如，一些研究人员研究了 540 名成年的被收养者的基因因素和家庭环境因素，发现这 540 名被收养者的体重和他们的亲生父母的体重之间有很高的相关性（Stunkard, et al. , 1986）。但是，这些被收养者的体重和他们养父母的体重之间却没有相关性。基于父母—子女的研究的另一个不足则是遗传性也可能被低估，因为孩子和父母在受到研究时处于不同的年龄段。如果不同的基因和/或环境因素对 BMI 指数的影响程度在不同的年龄段是不同的，那么父母—子女和兄弟姐妹之间的相关性会被减弱，遗传的影响就有可能被低估。此外，不同研究计算出的遗传度存在较大差异的原因可能是源于不同的研究设计类型（基于双胞胎的研究设计，基于家庭和收养家庭的研究设计等），小样本和研究对象年龄的不同（Beunen, et al. , 1998）。虽然这些研究都有一些不足，父母—子女和双胞胎研究仍然被广泛运用于遗传流行病学的研究中。这些研究也已经成功地表明了遗传是儿童性肥胖病因中最重要的影响因素之一。

## 二、基因对人体能量消耗的影响

肥胖的发生是源于能量摄入与能量消耗之间的不平衡。肥胖症的病因中，遗传是重要的因素之一，而遗传的影响其实包括了对能量消耗偏低的影响，和/或对能量摄入偏高的影响（Figueroa-Colon, et al. , 2000）。

（一）静息能量代谢

一个人总能量消耗的50% - 75%是以静息能量消耗（REE）的形式被消耗掉的（Ravussin & Bogardus, 1989）。个体之间REE的差异可能是导致肥胖症的原因之一。一些早期的研究表明肥胖父母的子女往往存在REE较低的问题，这可能导致儿童性肥胖（Griffiths & Payne, 1976; Griffiths, et al. , 1990）。有研究发现，11% REE的方差可以由遗传因素来解释（Bogardus, et al. , 1986）。另一项研究则发现，除去体脂率、年龄和性别的影响后，家庭遗传与能量消耗之间的组内相关系数为0. 26（Ravussin & Bogardus, 1989）。近期对静息能量消耗与肥胖的研究显示，当除去体格大小的影响后，REE 的遗传度系数为0. 3（X. Wu, et al. , 2004），除去甲状腺类激素和代谢风险的影响后，REE 的遗传系数为0. 29 ± 0. 08（Bosy-Westphal, et al. , 2008）。

但是，某些研究的数据并不支持肥胖父母的孩子REE会更低并且超重可能性更高的理论。比如，有研究发现，无论父母的体型是瘦或者胖，青春期前的女孩在24小时内无论是休息、睡觉或者进行一些体力活动的时候都有相近的能量消耗（Treuth, et al. , 2000）。另一项研究的结果显示，父亲和母亲中有一方肥胖的儿童调整后的平均REE要比那些父母都不肥胖的孩子低50卡路里/天，但这种情况没有在父亲和母亲都肥胖的孩子身上发现（Goran, et al.，1995）。有些研究人员指出没有发现低代谢率和超重之间关系的一个原因可能是，能引起超重的低代谢率也许被其他与肥胖相关的代谢风险因素给掩盖了（Bosy-Westphal，et al.，2008）。

（二）食物的热效应

食物的热效应（TEF）是由于进食引起能量消耗增加的现象。对 TEF 的研究已经持续了几十年。但是，TEF 对肥胖的发展是否有影响仍然不得而知。至今仅有个别对 TEF 的遗传度的研究被报道。其中一个研究的数据显示至少 40% - 50% TEF 的变化能由遗传来解释。TEF 的相关系数在异卵双胞胎、同卵双胞胎和父母—子女之间分别为 0.35、0.52 和 0.30（Bouchard，et al.，1989）。在另一项研究中，发现一般人进行亚极量强度训练运动时的 TEF 比肥胖者的 TEF 显著的高（Segal，et al.，1984）。这些研究显示肥胖父母的孩子更容易有低 TEF，这可能引起体重的增长。

（三）身体活动相关的能量消耗和总能量消耗

身体活动中的能量消耗（AEE）是总能量消耗中（TEE）的关键一项。一些研究显示人与人之间 AEE 和 TEE 的不同在一点程度上可以由遗传解释。比如，超重母亲生下的幼儿如果能量消耗减少，特别是身体活动减少会引起体重的快速增加（Roberts，et al.，1983）。另一项研究调查了 196 名非肥胖女生的能量消耗和体重状态，她们的能量消耗通过间接测功仪和双标水法分别进行测量，结果发现至少有一方父母体重超重的女生的 REE 和 TEE 数据和要高于其他女生（Bandini，et al.，2002）。

但是，另一项基于大量健康幼儿的研究并没有显示出幼儿的能量消耗与父母的体重水平相关（Davies, et al., 1995）。

### 三、遗传对能量摄入和食物喜好的影响

当能量摄入大于能量消耗时，即时是每天一点点，也可能引起儿童肥胖（Goran, 2001）。一项动物研究的结果显示，营养素的摄入在一定程度上受遗传影响（Reed, et al., 1997）。对儿童饮食习惯和食物喜好的研究也显示了类似的结果。研究发现孩子倾向于拒绝不熟悉的食物，并会慢慢体会出食物的口味与消化后结果之间的关系（Birch & Fisher, 1998）。除此之外，这项研究同样显示孩子会对食物的能量密度有反应，这也表明孩子的能量摄入和食物选择可能受到遗传的影响。

另一方面，一些对双胞胎的研究希望能确定遗传对能量摄入和食物喜好的影响。一项研究调查了1597名来自375个不同家庭的法裔研究对象三天的饮食记录（Perusse, et al., 1988）。但是，研究结果并没有显示出遗传对受测试的营养素摄入的显著影响（遗传度＜11%），这表明遗传因素可能不是影响孩子食物选择最主要的影响因素，而非遗传因素的影响可能是影响孩子食物摄入的主要影响因素。但仍然有一些研究显示了家庭因素对个人能量摄入和食物喜好的影响。比如，一项研究发现同卵双胞胎对不同类型食物的摄入的相似度超过了异卵双胞胎，该研究提示遗传对人们食物喜好存在影响（Heitmann, et al., 1999）。另一项典型的基于396对双胞胎的研究同样证明了遗传对孩子食物摄入的影响（Faith, et al., 2008）。

总的来说，对这些研究的回顾结果显示出了遗传和食物摄入之间的关联。虽然遗传的影响程度并不一定很高，但有越来越多的证据显示遗传在能量摄入和食物喜好方面起着很重要的作用，并可能增加肥胖的风险。

# 第三节　父母对儿童肥胖的认知、理念和知识

遗传是影响儿童期肥胖的因素之一，但可能并不是决定儿童期肥胖发展的最主要因素（Harrell, et al., 2001）。研究显示除了生物学和成长方面的因素，一系列心理学的、社会的、文化的以及环境上的因素也会影响孩子的食物摄入和身体活动（Sallis, et al., 1992）。对于那些想参与到儿童性肥胖预防的过程中的父母来说，父母对于子女体重状态的认知，对儿童期肥胖的理念以及对营养和运动的知识在儿童期肥胖的治疗中将起到很关键的作用。

## 一、父母对子女体重的认知

一些研究已经证明，青少年往往容易低估自己的体重（Skinner, et al., 2008）。那些对自己的体重有很清楚认识的青少年超重者或者肥胖者往往更愿意参与到控制体重的行为矫正活动中来（Bittner Fagan, et al., 2008）。一项在葡萄牙的研究发现，那些超重的孩子对于控制饮食的需要有着不正确的认识，对于自身健康状态的认知也较差（Fonseca & Gaspar de Matos, 2005）。但是，父母能否正确认识孩子的体重状态是个问题。另

一个问题是，与子女没有体重问题的父母相比，那些认识到子女体重问题的超重青少年的父母是否会更愿意帮助他们的子女控制体重。

不幸的是，大多数的研究显示父母往往低估了他们孩子体重问题的严重程度（Skinner, et al., 2008）。据报道，将近1/3的母亲低估了自己超重孩子的体重（Maynard, et al., 2003）。一个定性研究揭示，对于那些被定义为超重的学龄前儿童，父母往往都有着歪曲的理解，许多父母都不认为超重和肥胖是健康问题（Suzanne Goodell, et al., 2008）。这项研究同样显示，那些受教育程度不高的母亲更可能对她们孩子的体重状态认识错误（Baughcum, et al., 2000）。另一项研究同样显示，那些超重儿童或者面临超重危险的儿童的父母很少认为他们的子女超重或者担心子女体重超重的问题（Eckstein, et al., 2006）。

因此，在制定肥胖预防策略的时候或在一些体重管理项目中，人们需要考虑父母对于孩子体重错误认知的问题。此外，一些研究显示那些低估孩子体重的父母或者孩子本身，往往自身有比较差的饮食习惯，并且更难以养成健康的饮食习惯和运动习惯（Skinner, et al., 2008）。有一项研究调查了父母的心理反馈效应。在这项研究中，调查了伦敦6-11岁学龄儿童的体重和身高，并向他们的父母告知了孩子的体重状态。在向父母告知他们孩子体重的5周之前，这些父母的健康行为信息已经被记录下来，并在将孩子的体重信息反馈给他们的4周后，再次记录了这些父母的健康行为信息。研究发现孩子体重的反馈信息并没有影响那些正常体重儿童的父母的喂养子女的行为，但是对那些超重的女孩的父母来说，发现他们对孩子饮食的限制增加了（Grimmett, et al., 2008）。但是，另一项横断面研究显示对孩子体重的正确认识不一定能产生正面的影响，反而有可能产生一些负面的影响，比如强迫孩子节食（Neumark-Sztainer, et al., 2008）。这些相互矛盾的研究结果可能是由于不同的实验设计，特别是实验干预部分的设计，仍然需要更多的随机的或对照的干预研究来确定某种干预对孩子的体重管理是否有效。

## 二、父母对于运动及营养的理念和知识

有四类因素被发现对人们的饮食习惯有影响：收入，食物的价格，其他物品的价格和服务，口味、爱好和消费者对健康和营养的知识（Variyam & Blaylock, 1998）。因此，一般认为，有着良好营养学知识的父母更有可能为他们的子女选择健康的食物。一项英格兰的问卷调查中发现，营养知识最丰富的20%被调查者的饮食符合健康饮食指南的可能性是知识最不丰富的20%被调查者的25倍（Wardle, et al., 2000）。在另一项研究中发现，母亲的营养学知识和与健康饮食有关的看法，是影响孩子水果摄入（Gibson, et al., 1998）、纤维素摄入和低脂食物摄入（Variyam, et al., 1999）的重要因素之一。另一项研究则发现，虽然没有发现母亲的健康理念对学龄前儿童以及小学生的乳制品摄入习惯有任何影响，却发现与青少年的乳制品摄入量有关（Kim & Douthitt, 2003）。这种不一致的结果提示我们，父母们的营养知识对孩子在养成健康饮食习惯中起的作用可能不

是决定性的，但依然是重要的（Worsley，2002）。

增加儿童和青少年的身体活动的参与度是预防儿童期肥胖的重要手段之一。一些研究已经证明了对运动的知识是影响成人（Hagger，et al.，2002）和儿童（Trost，et al.，1997）运动量的因素之一。比如，一项纵向跟踪研究的结果显示知识程度一定程度上决定人的运动习惯（Rimal，2001）。另一项研究同样发现对怎样的运动强度能够保持健康和对坚持运动的理念与一个人的身体活动水平有关（Fitgerald，et al.，1994）。因此，父母们对运动的看法和知识对他们孩子的体力活动程度有着间接的影响。研究发现那些关心孩子身体活动程度的父母往往更愿意支持他们的孩子参与身体活动，比如，送孩子去参加体育活动等（Trost，et al.，2003）。但是，也有研究表明父母对运动看法与孩子的身体活动水平之间并没有关系（Kimiecik，et al.，1996）。另一项研究同样表明，知识和其他态度上的因素与肥胖之间的相关性要比身体活动相关行为的因素与肥胖之间的相关性低得多（Gordon-Larsen，2001）。即使如此，大多数的研究结果仍认为父母对营养和运动的知识和看法是预防儿童期肥胖的要素之一。

## 三、中国传统与父母对肥胖的认知、看法和知识

父母对肥胖的观念、看法和知识可能与文化价值观有关。有研究证明，对体重的不满意和节食的行为一定程度上与种族、文化有关（Altabe，1998；Gluck & Geliebter，2002）。在中国，一些对肥胖的传统观念和对营养和体力活动知识的缺乏与日渐增

多的儿童肥胖有关。比如，在中国的传统文化中，胖孩子往往被认为是健康孩子，好胃口也常常被认为是健康的表现（Y. N. Li，2008）。一项基于 140 名肥胖儿童的调查显示，36%的父亲和 28%的母亲没有意识到他们的孩子已经肥胖，一些父母甚至认为肥胖是健康的一种表现（Xiao, et al.，2001）。一项对中国父母肥胖知识的调查表明那些肥胖儿童的父母在测试中的分数比正常体重儿童的父母的分数更低（J. G. Wang, et al.，2007）。有一项目的在于增进父母对肥胖的理解和知识的干预性研究，干预前后收集的问卷数据显示父母对健康饮食的知识能通过干预来提高（Lv & Tian，2007）。这些研究的一项不足是这些调查问卷的发展过程和来源并没有被清楚地介绍，问卷的可靠性和有效性也没有得到验证。即便如此，这些研究仍然证明了在中国，父母对肥胖的认知、看法和知识可能与儿童期肥胖有关。

中国美食因其高超的制作技巧而闻名。但是在中国，大多数人更关心食物的颜色、香味、风味和食物的形状，较少关注食物的营养成分。因此，在中国家庭中，父母更关心的是食物的风味而不是食物所含的营养和热量（Y. N. Li，2008）。此外，许多中国成年人经历过贫穷的时代，这使得他们更倾向于为他们的孩子提供足够量的食物。在一项质化研究中，一些中国受访者诉说由于在 1940 年到 1970 年之间，他们经历了极度的饥饿和贫穷，这种悲惨的经历导致他们经常担心他们的子女会吃不到足够的食物，因而会倾向于向他们的子女提供超过子女需要的食物量（Jiang, et al.，2007）。

在中国的传统中，儿童在学校的学业表现是中国父母最关注的事情。需要指出的是，教育是在中国大陆获得个人提升最重要的途径之一（Xiang, et al., 1997）。因此，包括身体活动在内的任何可能影响子女学业的事物，都可能不受他们父母的支持。比如，有研究调查了参加中学田径队的学生运动员。结果发现，虽然大部分父母都认为体育训练有益于子女的健康和体质，但是大部分学生父母并不支持他们的子女参加校队训练，因为训练可能占用子女大量时间，可能对他们的学习成绩造成负面影响（C. L. Li & Li, 2005）。另一项香港的研究也发现，香港地区儒家思想和后殖民主义的交互影响可能是体育和身体活动在香港家庭中处于次要地位的重要原因（Ha, et al., 2010）。

综上所述，仅有少量的研究调查了中国父母对于子女饮食、运动和肥胖问题的认知、理念和知识。这些研究结果表明父母对于子女饮食、运动和肥胖问题的认知、理念和知识可能受到中国传统文化的影响。还需要更多的研究来倡导中国儿童健康饮食和进行充足的身体活动。

## 第四节　父母教养子女的行为

### 一、父母教养子女的行为和子女的食物摄入

儿童的饮食是引起儿童肥胖最重要的环境因素之一（Birch & Fisher, 1998），会受到父母、朋友、媒体和他们自身口味和偏好的影响（Golan & Crow, 2004a; Lindsay, et al., 2006）。对儿

童饮食影响最大的父母教养子女的行为应该是父母喂养子女行为，具体包括限制饮食、鼓励或强迫子女饮食、把食物当作奖励等。父母喂养子女的行为会影响子女的饮食习惯和食物偏好，子女自身对于饮食摄入的控制，并最终影响他们的体重水平（Nguyen，et al. 1996）。有研究综述调查了 22 项关于父母喂养子女的行为与子女能量摄入、体重水平关系的研究（Faith，Scanlon，et al.，2004）。结果显示，虽然研究的方法和结果不尽相同，但是其中 19 项研究（86%）报道了至少一种父母喂养子女的行为与子女体重水平存在相关。因此，父母喂养子女的方法是影响儿童肥胖发展的重要因素。

**饮食限制**

针对儿童肥胖最为常用的父母喂养子女的行为是限制饮食的分量和限制不健康饮食。采用这种喂养行为的父母可能认为他们这么做对于子女健康是有益的。但是这种假设并没有得到近年来研究数据的支持。有研究通过观察法调查了限制儿童食用某种美味零食的效果。该研究发现，与另一种类似的未受限制的零食相比，儿童经过五周的限制后对受限零食表现出了更多的兴趣（Fisher & Birch，1999b）。一项纵向跟踪研究则显示，父母限制女儿饮食可能反而导致女儿养成在不饿的情况吃零食的饮食习惯（Fisher & Birch，2002）。另一项纵向跟踪研究还发现，在控制了子女 3 岁时的 BMI 的情况下，父母在子女 5 岁时限制子女饮食的行为可能导致子女在 7 岁时体重水平更高（Faith，Berkowitz，et al.，2004）。

几位研究者提出了父母限制子女饮食行为与子女体重水平

相关的可能机制。研究者们认为，限制儿童吃某种食物反而会激起儿童对此种食品的注意，因而增加他们得到和吃这种食物的欲望（Fisher & Birch, 1999b）。因此，在短期内，父母限制子女饮食的方法可以减少子女不健康食品的数量，降低总热量的摄入。但是，当子女们摆脱父母控制时就会尽可能地去吃这些被父母限制的食品。一项观察性研究也证明了该假设（Klesges, et al., 1991）。在该研究中，当儿童们被允许从几十种食物中自由选择食物时，他们选择了大量的不健康食品，这些食品25%的热量来自添加的糖。但是，当孩子们知道他们父母会来检查他们选什么食品时，孩子们会减少他们挑选的食物，或者少挑一些不健康的食物。

鉴于已经有一些研究证明了限制饮食的方法可能存在一些负面效应，这种喂养子女的行为不应该推荐给父母。近年来的研究结果提示，应该向父母，特别是向那些关心子女体重水平的父母提供喂养子女方法和技术方面的信息和指导（Clark, et al., 2007）。

### 鼓励或强迫饮食

父母常常使用的喂养子女的另一个行为是鼓励或强迫饮食，也就是不许子女剩饭或要求子女吃某些食物。有研究表明这种喂养子女的方法有助于提高子女对蔬菜和水果的摄入量（Bourcier, et al., 2003）。还有的研究发现，父母鼓励或强迫子女饮食的行为与儿童的脂肪总量可能存在负相关（Spruijt-Metz, et al., 2002）。另一项基于大学生记忆的研究则表明父母鼓励或强迫子女饮食的行为可能导致子女对于该种食物长期的负面回忆（Batsell，et al.，2002）。

进一步研究儿童对父母鼓励或强迫饮食行为的反应可能有助于我们进一步理解父母鼓励或强迫饮食行为对于子女体重水平的影响。有研究发现，与不胖的母亲相比，胖妈妈更愿意采用鼓励或强迫子女饮食的行为，特别是对一些新奇的食物（Lumeng & Burke，2006）。在该研究中比较有趣的一个现象是，与熟悉的食物相比，胖妈妈们会更频繁地鼓励子女吃新奇的食品。

综上所述，各类相关研究的结果还存在较大差异，这也提示鼓励或强迫子女饮食与儿童体重水平的关系可能要比它看起来更复杂。鼓励或强迫子女吃某种食物可以增加其对该种食物的摄入量。但是，从长远来看，这种行为可能导致子女对该食物留下负面印象。

**以食物作为奖励**

用食物来影响儿童的行为也是父母常常采用的喂养子女的行为。一项针对低收入母亲喂养子女行为的调查显示，食物不仅仅是母亲们为子女提供能量和营养的物品，还是他们鼓励子女表现好的奖励品（Baughcum，et al.，1998）。一般认为，采用这种方式鼓励子女表现好，会让子女在不饿的情况下吃东西，从而会影响儿童自我感知饱和饿的能力。一项实验研究发现，用某种食物作为奖励子女表现好的方法会加强儿童对该种食物的偏爱（Birch，et al.，1980）。如果长期使用这种父母教养子女的行为，可能对儿童能量摄入自我调整的能力产生负面影响，导致儿童在决定吃多少东西时仍过多地依赖外部的信号而不是自身的感觉（Rhee，2008）。因此，这种父母教养子女的行为可能导致儿童摄入了大大超过他们自身需要的热量。

在关于父母教养子女的行为和儿童饮食习惯的相关研究中需要注意几个问题。首先，一些研究发现父母喂养子女的行为和儿童体重水平的关系是双向的，但是横断面研究并不能确定这种关系的因果关系（Clark，et al.，2007；Faith，Berkowitz，et al.，2004）。比如，假如子女的体重超重了，父母可能会限制子女接触不健康食品。但是，儿童也可能因为父母采用了限制不健康饮食的原因而体型较瘦。这可能就是一些横断面调查不能发现父母喂养子女的行为与子女体重水平相关关系的可能原因之一（Baughcum，et al.，1998；Saelens，et al.，2000）。

另一个可能影响父母喂养子女行为的因素是社会经济地位。一项质化研究在一些社会经济地位较低的母亲中发现了母亲喂养子女的理念和行为可能与儿童肥胖有关（Baughcum，et al.，1998）。比如，该研究发现，社会经济地位较低的母亲更愿意用食物来改变他们子女的行为。另一项研究则发现，教育水平较低的母亲更倾向于鼓励或者强迫她们的子女多吃（Lumeng & Burke，2006）。因此，这些研究也提示，还需要更多的研究工作探索适应于不同社会经济阶层的有效干预方案。

综上所述，不同的父母喂养子女的行为可能与儿童肥胖的发生有关。目前的研究建议，让儿童在一个更自然的环境中成长，由父母来决定子女吃什么，什么时候吃、在哪里吃、吃还是不吃、吃多少的问题则应让子女自己决定（Satter，2004）。

（一）父母的榜样作用和儿童饮食摄入

另一种可能影响子女饮食习惯的父母教养子女的行为是通过父母的榜样作用或观察学习。一项基于实验室的研究发现，当给儿童吃一种新的食物时，当儿童看到别人在吃同样食物时会更愿意吃这种食物，但是当他仅仅看到有其他人或者看到别人在吃其他食物时，吃这种新食物的可能性相比前种情况更低（Addessi，et al.，2005）。因此，有学者提出了假说，父母通过在子女面前吃健康食品并向子女表示他们喜欢这种食物，可能可以影响他们子女的饮食行为（Golan & Crow，2004a；Lindsay，et al.，2006）。有一些研究也证明了该假说。有研究证明了父母和子女的许多食物的摄入量存在中度相关（$r < 0.50$）（Oliveria，et al.，1992）。父母以身作则的健康饮食行为频率对于儿童饮食习惯的发展具有长期的影响（Tibbs，et al.，2001）。另一项研究也发现，父母自己吃蔬菜水果也可以带动他们女儿多吃蔬菜水果，以增加营养素的摄入，减少脂肪的摄入（Fisher，et al.，2002）。当青少年长大后，他们会逐渐受到他们的朋友越来越多的影响。但是，研究发现在非洲裔家庭的青少年中，家庭在提供支持方面仍然扮演着重要的作用（Wilson & Ampey-Thornhill，2001）。通过这些研究，我们发现父母可以间接地通过榜样效应塑造他们子女的行为。因此，在儿童肥胖的干预过程中，建议父母自身也采纳健康的行为以更好地改变他们子女的饮食行为。

## 二、父母教养子女的行为与儿童身体活动水平

目前的身体活动指南建议，儿童应在每周的大部分天数，

最好是每天，进行至少60分钟身体活动。但是，目前大部分儿童未能达到每天60分钟身体活动的推荐量（Nicklas, et al., 2008）。体育运动或身体活动的参与是一个复杂的行为，受到多方面因素的影响。学校被认为在增加儿童青少年身体活动方面起着核心作用（Pate, et al., 2006）。但是，是儿童的父母来决定子女是否走路去上学，决定子女骑自行车的距离，帮助子女参加舞蹈、游泳等课外活动。因此，父母在子女参与身体活动上也起着非常重要的作用（Mulvihill, et al., 2000）。

父母支持他们的子女参与身体活动有多种形式。支持的形式包括购买运动服装和运动装备、开车接送子女去运动场、鼓励子女参与身体活动、自身经常做运动作为榜样（Prochaska, et al., 2002）。有研究帮助归纳了几种主要的父母教养子女的方式：接纳和社会支持、自身的榜样效应、对子女的期望、通过奖励和惩罚强化相关行为、给予详细的指导（Woolger & Power, 1993）。

（一）榜样作用

影响儿童身体活动最重要的父母教养子女的行为之一是榜样作用。Framingham 儿童研究的数据显示，与不积极参与身体活动父母的子女相比，积极参与身体活动父母的子女积极投身身体活动的可能性更大。而且，与父母双方都不积极参与身体活动的儿童相比，父母双方都积极参与身体活动的儿童积极投身身体活动的可能性是前者的5.8倍（Moore, et al., 1991）。一项来自挪威的调查则发现，青少年参与体育活动受到他们家庭成员和朋友是否参与体育活动影响，而且两者的相互关系主要是基于儿童与身体活动量充足家庭成员的关系（Skille，2005）。这一系列研究表明，父母和子女身体活动水平相关的可能原因之一是父母的榜样作用。一项质化研究也发现，父母的榜样作用是提高青少年身体活动量最重要的方法之一（Wright，et al.，2008）。综上所述，这些研究清楚地表明父母的榜样作用会影响子女的身体活动水平。

（二）父母的支持

有几篇研究综述总结了关于父母支持与子女身体活动关系的研究（Sallis，et al.，2000；van der Horst，Paw，et al.，2007）。遗憾的是，这些研究也没有定论。比如，有一些研究发现，得到父母更多支持的儿童会更积极地参与体育活动（O'Loughlin，et al.，1999）。另一项研究则发现，得到父母鼓励的青少年每周积极参加体育活动的天数比没有得到父母鼓励的青少年多（King，et al.，2008）。但是，也有研究的结果显示，父母的支持并不是与客观测量的身体活动水平相关的因素（Sallis，et al.，2002）。还有研究发现，父母自我报告的支持可能与女孩的身体活动量相关，但不具有统计学意义（$r = 0.26$，$p < 0.06$）。但另一项分别由自我报告和加速器测量两种方式测量身体活动的研究则发现，父母的支持与青少年自我报告的身体活动相关，但是研究者未发现父母支持和加速器测量的身体活动水平相关（Prochaska，et al.，2002）。

综上所述，目前对于父母支持和儿童身体活动水平的研究结果不太一致。研究结果不一致的原因可能包括：身体活动测量方法存在差异、样本特点存在差异、统计分析方法存在差异

（van der Horst, Paw, et al., 2007）。比如，有的研究采用问卷的方式调查受试对象的身体活动水平，有的研究则采用客观的测量方法（如计步器、加速器等）。有的研究招募的是超重或具有超重风险的研究对象，而有的研究的研究对象则是正常体重的儿童。因此，还需要更多的研究进一步确定父母支持与儿童身体活动水平的关系。

## 三、父母教养子女的行为和中国儿童肥胖

来自西方国家的研究已经证明了父母教养子女的行为与儿童肥胖存在联系。鉴于中国的社会结构和传统文化与西方国家存在的差异，中国父母教养子女的行为比如喂养子女的行为和父母对青少年身体活动的支持也可能与西方国家父母的行为有所不同。

"鼓励或强迫子女饮食"被认为是西方国家父母最常用的喂养子女行为之一（Bourcier, et al., 2003；Spruijt-Metz, et al., 2002）。研究发现，这种喂养子女的行为在中国父母中也普遍使用。不过，大部分中国父母选择提醒而不是强迫他们的子女吃东西。有调查发现有56%常常提醒子女吃他们认为健康的食品，还有7.7%的父母会强迫他们吃这些食物（W. J. Ma, et al., 2001）。有一项在欧美国家很少被报道而在中国非常常见的父母教养子女的行为是"在吃饭的时候批评子女"。分别有14.8%和27.5%的父母常常或有时在吃饭的时候批评子女，这将导致有5.6%的儿童在吃饭时一点东西都没吃（W. J. Ma, et al., 2001）。此外，一项针对北京市930户有2-6岁儿童家庭的调

查发现，父母和子女的饮食习惯、看电视和身体活动之间存在很强的相关（Jiang，et al.，2006）。

我国的研究也显示，父母可能通过榜样作用、提供经济上和情感上的支持来影响儿童的身体活动（C. Sun，et al.，2008）。比如，一项有1614名中学生参与的横断面调查显示，身体活动积极的父母的子女积极参与身体活动的可能性也更大（Y. H. Sun，et al.，1994）。另一项来自香港104名超重儿童父母的研究也发现，父亲的榜样作用与子女的身体活动存在相关，且相关具有显著性（Lau，et al.，2007）。

虽然目前已经有一些颇具价值的针对父母教养子女的行为对儿童肥胖影响的研究，但是需要指出的是，这些研究还存在一些局限性。比如，父母教养子女的行为可能受到文化因素影响，中国的父母可能具有一些中国特色的教养子女的行为。如，中国父母常常喜欢在吃饭的时候给子女夹菜以表达他们对子女的爱。这种行为有可能影响子女自身调节能量摄入的能力。但是，这些中国父母传统的教养子女的行为与子女体重水平的关系却没有进行深入研究。目前很少有研究深入对比了中国父母与西方国家父母在教养子女的行为方面的差异。尽管如此，我国这些研究也已经成功地证明了父母教养子女的行为与子女体重水平存在相关。

## 第五节　父母教养子女的方式

父母教养子女的行为是描述父母做了什么，而父母教养子女的方式则是指父母如何做的。父母教养子女的方式被定义为父母教养子女行为表达和被子女解读的情感背景（Rhee, 2008）。因此，父母教养子女的方式不仅将影响父母对于子女饮食和运动的行为，还可能影响子女们身体活动、饮食习惯、情感，并最终影响子女超重和肥胖的风险。因而，与仅仅注重父母教养子女的行为的干预方式相比，同时注重父母教养子女的行为和方式的儿童肥胖干预更为有效（Rhee, et al. , 2006）。

## 一、父母教养子女方式的理论框架

目前应用最多的父母教养子女方式的相关理论是 Baumrind 建立的，该理论将父母教养子女方式分成两个维度：关爱和控制（Baumrind, 1971）。以两个维度上的量和质为出发点，可以把父母分成四种教养方式，民主型（高关爱、高控制）、专制型（低关爱、高控制）、溺爱型（高关爱、低控制）与放任型（低关爱、低控制）（Darling & Steinberg, 1993）。

## 二、父母教养子女方式对子女的影响

民主型教养方式被认为是最好的父母教养子女的方式，研究也发现该种教养方式有助于提高子女各方面的表现。相反，另外三种父母教养子女的方式不能满足子女发展的需求，因此可能导致子女在某些方面表现不佳。比如，有研究发现，父母教养子女的方式可能会影响青少年的学业成绩和表现（Aunola, et al. , 2000）。另一项研究则发现，民主型的父母能够更成功地让子女远离吸食毒品问题（Baumrind, 1991）。

一些研究则报道了父母教养子女的行为与儿童体重水平的关系。一项针对澳大利亚4983名4－5岁儿童的纵向跟踪研究显示，与民主型父亲的子女相比，溺爱型和放任型父亲的子女在高BMI组别的几率更高（Wake, et al., 2007）。另一项研究则发现，与民主型母亲的子女相比，专制型、溺爱型和放任型母亲的子女出现超重问题的可能性更大（Rhee, et al., 2006）。针对拉丁裔父母及其子女的调查也发现，子女的健康饮食和身体活动与父母积极的鼓励和监管有关，而且父母更严苛的教养子女的方式更有助于子女保持饮食健康；但是父母过度的控制则可能导致子女饮食不健康（Arredondo, et al., 2006）。

## 三、中国父母教养子女的方式与儿童肥胖

在欧美国家，已经建立了父母教养子女方式的理论和模型。但是许多研究者都提出一个重要的研究问题"不同文化背景下父母们教养子女的方式是否有差异？"。Chao认为用专制和民主来形容中国父母教养子女的方式并没有抓住中国父母教养子女方式的特点，可能不太符合中国父母的特征。Chao也是第一个在国际相关文献中采用"管"来表达父母教养子女方式的学者（Chao, 1994）。在过去的2000年中，儒家思想在中国的传统教育中占据非常重要的地位。虽然，在最近30年，中国社会受到西方文化强烈的冲击，但是大部分中国人的理念、行为和教养子女的方式都深受儒家思想影响（Holroyd, 2003；P. Wu, et al., 2002；Xu, et al., 2005）。中国人教养子女的方式常常被世人认

为是"专制"、"严格"和"高控制"的（Lin & Fu, 1990；Steinberg, et al., 1992）。事实上，传统的儒家思想对家庭成员间的关系进行了规定。在传统的中国家庭，子女需要严格服从和尊重他们的父母（Bond & Hwang, 1986）。研究也发现，美国人更注重人自身的能力和天赋，而中国人则更强调高度的自律、服从父母、父母的高度参与，这些理念都是植根于中国传统文化（Chao, 1994；F. M. Chen & Luster, 2002）。

研究发现，中国父母教养子女的方式深受儒家思想影响，而这种教养子女的方式也影响着子女在学业和社会中的表现（X. Y. Chen, et al., 1997；Nelson, et al., 2006），也与子女的性格有关（Porter, et al., 2005）。但是，目前仅有非常少的几项研究对中国父母教养子女的行为、方式和子女体重水平关系进行了研究。比如，有一项基于163名华裔8－10岁儿童和他们母亲的横向调查显示民主型父母教养子女的方式与儿童BMI存在正相关（J. L. Chen & Kennedy, 2004）。另一项来自香港的研究则发现，父母的影响，特别是父亲的榜样作用，可以显著地影响子女对体育运动的态度（Lau, et al., 2007）。

另一方面，中国施行独生子女政策后，不仅让中国自然人口出生率大大降低（Jing, 1994），还改变了数以万计父母教养子女的行为和方式。在过去的30年中，由于许多中国家庭中仅有一个孩子，许多孩子都被他们的父母和其他家庭成员宠坏了。此外，在中国传统文化中，中国父亲和母亲在家庭中扮演的角色有所不同，父亲被认为应该是"严"的，而母亲被认为应该是"慈"的（Berndt, et al., 1993）。但是，目前还没有研究报道中国父亲和母亲教养子女的方式对子女体重水平的影响是否也有区别，还需要进一步的研究探索中国父母教养子女的方式与儿童肥胖的关系。

总而言之，在过去的 30 年，中国父母教养子女的方式受到了中国传统文化和西方文化的影响。虽然，有研究报道了中国和美国父母教养子女方式的差异，但是目前中国父母教养子女方式的相关理论还不够完善。此外，基于美国父母的父母教养子女方式的理论（Baumrind，1971），也广泛地应用于中国父母教养子女方式的研究（X. Y. Chen，et al.，1997；Pong，et al.，2009；Porter，et al.，2005），这也提示我们这一理论仍可以用于解决关于中国父母的研究问题。

# 第六节　家庭环境

## 一、食物的供应情况和易得性

父母可以通过改变家庭的环境来影响子女的体重水平。有这样一个动物实验：两组老鼠，分别被提供了 5 瓶饲料加 1 瓶水和 5 瓶水加 1 瓶饲料（饲料和水被消耗后会及时补充），经过一段时间后，被提供了 5 瓶饲料加 1 瓶水的一组老鼠要比被提供了 5 瓶水加 1 瓶饲料的老鼠胖。这一项实验提示，不健康饮食和肥胖问题最主要的原因是食物的供应而不是某些生理机制（Tordoff，2002）。而这一研究同时也提示，在儿童肥胖的干预中，需要考虑到家里食物的易得性问题。

最近的一些研究发现，食物的供应情况是影响儿童蔬菜和水果摄入量最重要的因素之一（Blanchette & Brug, 2005）。比如，有几项横断面调查发现，家里水果和蔬菜的供应情况可以预测儿童蔬菜水果的摄入量（Cullen, et al., 2003；Neumark-Sztainer, et al., 2003）。另一方面，缺乏安全而富含营养的食物会增加患肥胖症和其他健康问题的风险（Adams, et al., 2003）。一项纵向研究也发现，家庭蔬菜和水果的供应情况是影响蔬菜水果摄入量的重要因素之一（Larson, et al., 2007）。此外，不仅仅食物的供应情况，食物的易得性也会影响儿童的饮食。比如，有研究发现，假如将胡萝卜切成小块，并放在儿童可以接触到的范围内，可以增加儿童吃胡萝卜的可能性。因此，要增加子女健康食品的摄入量，父母应该增加健康食物的供应量，增强健康食品的易得性。

还有研究证实了快餐食品的供应得越多，肥胖的发生率也越高（Jeffery & French, 1998），因此家长除了要增加健康食品的易得性和供应量，还需要通过减少家中不健康食品的供应量，从而控制子女非健康食品的摄入量。虽然也有研究发现，限制儿童吃某种食物可能激起儿童对被禁食物的关注，反而增加儿童对这类食物的食欲（Fisher & Birch, 1999b），但是大部分针对减肥的成功行为干预方案都需要限制家中不健康食品的供应（Young, et al., 2007）。因此，尽管存在一些负面效应，还是建议父母控制肥胖或超重儿童不健康食品的摄入（Hughes, et al., 2008）。

## 二、家庭和社区身体活动的环境

### (一)健身器材

父母可以通过多种形式促进儿童积极参与身体活动。有研究发现，儿童家中的运动器材数量与他们的身体活动水平呈正比（Dunton, et al., 2003）。还有的研究发现，女孩们身体活动量与她们自己认为的家中运动器械多少有关（Motl, et al., 2007）。不过，也有一些研究数据发现客观测量的女孩的中等强度身体活动与家里的运动器械不存在显著相关（Trost, et al., 1999）。另一项研究则报道，在横断面研究中家里的运动器械对身体活动量存在影响，而在纵向跟踪研究中则没有发现这种效应（Motl, et al., 2005）。总而言之，虽然家中运动器械的多少可能不是影响儿童肥胖的主要因素，但是还是建议在儿童肥胖的干预中考虑运动器械的因素。

### (二)家庭和社区的身体活动环境

关于建筑环境对于肥胖影响的研究显示，生活在高密度、高道路连通性、土地综合利用的社区居民比低密度、道路连通性差、土地利用单一的社区居民更积极地参与身体活动（步行或骑自行车）（Saelens, et al., 2003）。此外，到运动和休闲场所的距离、人行道、快餐店的距离、快餐店的数量等都被发现与社区居民肥胖的发展有关（Papas, et al., 2007）。但是目前大部分研究均是基于成年人的研究。近 10 年来，建筑环境对儿童肥胖的影响也引起了学术界的关注。比如，有研究发现，是否具有运动场所与儿童特别是女孩的中等、剧烈的身体活动水平有关（Zask, et al., 2001）。另一项研究则发现，步行环境不佳的社区居民比步行环境较好的社区居民有更高的 BMI，也更容易出现体重超重问题（Saelens, et al., 2003）。此外，来自中国的研究也发现，居住小区附近没有人行道的儿童身体活动不足的可能性更大（M. Li, et al., 2006）。不过，也有的研究发现，到运动场地的距离、到快餐店的距离、社区的犯罪率与人们的超重并不相关（Burdette & Whitaker, 2004）。

社区安全问题是另一项可能影响父母对于儿童身体活动态度的因素。许多儿童抱怨，因为某些安全问题（如，穿越交通繁忙的马路等），他们的父母不让他们骑车出门或在远离家门的地方玩耍（Mulvihill, et al., 2000）。有研究调查了可能影响父母选择子女玩耍地点的因素（Sallis, et al., 1997）。结果显示，安全问题是父母们最关心的问题之一。但是，一项在美国 20 个大城市的横断面调查发现，母亲感受到的社区安全与他们的子女在屏幕前的时间（看电视、用电脑等时间）相关，但与他们的子女户外玩耍的时间以及发生肥胖的风险不存在相关（Burdette & Whitaker, 2005）。另一项研究也发现，受试对象感受到的社区安全与自我报告的身体活动水平不存在直接或间接的相关（Motl, et al., 2007）。

总之，虽然有一些研究认为建筑环境可能与人们的身体活动不存在具有统计意义的相关，但是许多研究结果仍表明，家庭和社区的环境是影响儿童身体活动的重要因素（Franzini, et al., 2009）。

# 第七节　其他因素

## 一、儿童的年龄和敏感期

在儿童肥胖的发展过程中存在几个敏感期为肥胖的预防和干预提供了机会窗口，因此这几个时间段也是父母影响儿童肥胖的关键时期。儿童认知发展的关键期也可能是儿童肥胖预防中行为改变的最有效的时期。研究者们确定了几个儿童肥胖发展中可能的关键期或敏感期（Dietz，1994）。

母亲的怀孕期可能是干预的敏感期之一。有研究发现，婴儿在母亲怀孕的早期如果出现过急性的营养不良问题，则在其后面的生命周期中可能更容易出现超重问题（Strauss，1997）。基于动物模型的研究则显示，小动物在母亲怀孕前两周的营养状况将决定其在断奶后早期的能量利用的控制能力（Anguita，et al.，1993）。此外，其他一些研究则发现，母亲在怀孕期间吸烟可能是导致子女肥胖的危险因素之一（Toschke，et al.，2003；Von Kries，et al.，2002）。而母亲在怀孕期患糖尿病也被发现与儿童肥胖有关（Dabelea，et al.，2008）。因此，关于儿童肥胖预防中的一项重要策略是，在母亲怀孕期应戒烟并避免糖尿病问题。虽然，怀孕期的因素可能对儿童的 BMI 影响的比例不高（Smith，et al.，2007），但是怀孕期仍是儿童肥胖发展的敏感期。

儿童们建立饮食习惯基础以及为一生打下营养基础的婴儿期（Westenhoefer，2002），是父母应该关注的儿童肥胖发展的另一个敏感期。在这个阶段，许多研究都在关注母乳喂养是否与儿童肥胖有关。比如，有研究发现，母乳喂养的时间超过6个月可能有助于预防儿童肥胖（Toschke, et al., 2007）。一项来自德国的横断面研究发现母乳喂养是肥胖发展的重要保护性因素。母乳喂养具有的保护性效应的可能机制是，与使用奶瓶喂养婴儿相比，母乳喂养可以帮助婴儿学习如何调节他们的能量摄入（Lindsay, et al., 2006）。不过，一项来自英国的基于1958年出生的受试对象的跟踪研究则没有发现母乳喂养与儿童期BMI存在联系（Parsons, et al., 2003）。该研究发现，母乳喂养是保护成年人BMI升高的保护性因素，但是这种影响在控制了一些变量后（父母体重水平、社会经济地位等）消失了或不再具有统计学意义了。另一项近期的研究也不支持母乳运动与减少儿童肥胖存在联系（Kramer, et al., 2008）。虽然，关于母乳喂养对于儿童肥胖影响的研究结果仍不一致，研究者们仍建议父母应完全母乳喂养子女6个月，同时母乳加辅食的周期应坚持至少两年（Hoddinott, et al., 2008）。

在儿童的身体活动和饮食习惯逐渐向成人靠拢，并逐渐养成自身的饮食和运动习惯的儿童成长早期，也是父母影响儿童肥胖的几个重要敏感期之一。虽然儿童早期的学习过程受到先天因素影响（Birch & Fisher, 1998），但是后天的学习对于儿童食物选择的发展仍是非常重要的（Westenhoefer, 2002）。不过，随着儿童长大，父母对于儿童肥胖的影响也在逐渐减弱。比如有研究发现，父母肥胖显著地增加了10岁以下肥胖子女和非肥胖子女成年后肥胖的风险。而对于10岁以上的儿童而言，无论父母胖或不胖，儿童期的体重水平才是成年后肥拌的最重要影响因素（Whitaker, et al., 1997）。另一项研究则建议，肥胖父母的 3 - 9 岁肥胖儿童是最好的接受干预对象，因为父母们仍有机会在子女的儿童早期塑造和改变他们子女的行为（Epstein, et al., 1990）。但是，在 10 岁以后，父母对于子女体重问题的影响就显著地下降了。

## 二、社会经济地位

主要是由父母的收入、教育和职业所决定的家庭社会经济地位，可能是影响父母对儿童肥胖作用的另一项因素之一。不难想象，社会经济地位较低的父母购买新鲜蔬菜水果、高质量运动器械、运动服装的可能性较低，也不太可能提供安全而适合步行的家庭周边环境给他们的子女。事实上，社会经济地位是影响儿童肥胖的重要因素之一已经得到了广泛认同，但是在发达国家和发展中国家，肥胖与社会经济地位的关系可能有所不同。比如，在美国，社会经济地位较高的青少年肥胖或超重的概率较低。相反，在中国，则是社会经济地位较低的青少年肥胖或超重的概率较低（Y. Wang, 2001）。目前的研究认为，在发达国家，社会经济地位较低的人群比社会经济地位较高的人群更容易出现肥胖，而在发展中国家，社会经济地位较低的人群的肥胖比例比社会经济地位较高的人群低（McLaren, 2007; Y. Wang, 2001）。另外，社会经济地位与儿童肥胖的关系在不同的种族中可能有所不同（Whitaker & Orzol, 2006）。最近的研究显示，社会经济地位与青少年肥胖的负相关仅限于白人儿童，而在黑人儿童青少年中没有发现（Y. Wang & Zhang, 2006）。不过，大部分关于社会经济地位的研究为横断面调查，并不能证明社会经济地位与肥胖风险之间的长期因果关系。基于发达国家的几项纵向跟踪研究则调查了成年人社会经济地位与体重变化的关系（Ball & Crawford, 2005b）。还需要更多的针对儿童，特别是发展中国家儿童的纵向跟踪研究对已有研究加以证实。总体而言，目前的研究发现，儿童肥胖可能受到家庭社会经济地位影响，但是肥胖与社会经济地位的关系在不同的国家、不同种族会有所不同。

目前对于社会经济地位与肥胖发展相互关系的机制尚未研究清楚。一些研究提出了一些可能的机制。比如，在发展中国家，社会经济地位低的人群肥胖率也更低的主要原因被认为是与食物缺乏、体力劳动中能量消耗较大等原因有关。发展中国家社会经济地位高的人群肥胖率高的原因则被归结于充足的食物供应，以及特殊文化环境下对于体型的不同解读（Sobal & Stunkard, 1989）。而在发达国家，研究者们则试图从行为的角度进行调查。总结下来，可能的调节因素包括：社会经济地位低的家长们缺乏身体活动和营养相关知识、缺乏行为技巧、对于肥胖不同的标准、贫民区不易买到健康食品等（Ball & Crawford, 2005b）。比如，有研究发现，不同的社会经济地位阶层所具有的营养知识有显著差别，而且教育水平越低、社会地位越低，所具有的营养知识也越少（Parmenter, et al., 2000）。另一项研究则发现社会经济地位与能量的摄入量呈反比，而社会经济地位与对体重的关注、所获得的健康饮食和身体活动相关的社会支持呈正比（Jeffery & French, 1996）。还有研究者建立了一个理论模型，该模型解释了人们在饮食摄入、运动上的社会文化的差异，而这种差异最终体现在体重上（Ball & Crawford, 2005a）。不过，有研究也发现，由社会经济地位差异所引起的人们在行为上的差异并不能完全解释不同社会经济地位的人在体重上的差异（Ball, et al., 2003）。因此，还需要进一步的研究来解释社会经济地位影响儿童肥胖的其他可能机制。

# 第八节 干 预

许多研究都已经证明了在儿童减肥项目中父母的参与非常重要，因而在儿童肥胖的防治指南中强调了父母参与和支持的重要性（Barlow & the Expert Committee, 2007）。许多专家指出，假如两名父母甚至是有一名父母没有参与到儿童肥胖的干预中，这样的干预就不太可能取得成功（Dietz & Robinson, 2005）。

基于学校、基于家庭和基于社区的干预是三种最常用的儿童肥胖干预方法。在许多研究中，通过父母的干预往往是一个全面干预方案的一小部分（Lindsay, et al., 2006）。大部分这些综合性干预在儿童肥胖治疗上都取得了不错的效果（Foster, et al., 2008；Robertson, et al., 2008）。一项长达10年的纵向跟踪研究发现，对肥胖儿童和父母都进行干预的方案要比单独对肥胖儿童进行干预的方案效果更好（Epstein, et al., 1990）。一个系统性综述也发现，教给父母和儿童越多的行为矫正技巧，减体重的干预成功率就越高（McLean, et al., 2003）。但是，这些干预方案都是综合性的干预，综合了针对儿童、老师、同学、父母及其他家庭成员的干预，因此也无法厘清针对父母的干预是否取得了实际效果。

最近，有人提出了一项结合了行为、社会学习以及家庭系统的特殊儿童肥胖干预方案（Golan & Weizman, 2001）。该方案以父母（而不是肥胖儿童）为干预对象，强调健康生活方式而不是单纯降体重。这种仅仅针对父母的干预具有的一个优点是，避免了传统干预方式的负面心理影响。比如，针对肥胖的干预有时不仅仅是干预儿童的食物摄入和身体活动，还可能导致儿童因为参加减肥训练而产生羞耻感，以及可能被其他孩子嘲笑而不合群（Sjoberg, et al. , 2005）。而单独针对父母而不是儿童的干预方案则可以避免这些问题。

另一方面，对这些只针对父母的干预方案的第 1 年、第 2 年和第 7 年的跟踪回访的结果也显示，与传统的干预方式相比，单独针对父母的干预方案让肥胖儿童减了更多的体重（Golan & Crow, 2004b）。采用单独针对父母的干预方案，通过多方面的父母健康教育进行干预的可行性也得到了证实（McGarvey, et al. , 2004）。此外，其他一些类似的研究采用相似的理念也都取得了巨大的成功。比如，有一个研究发现，超重或肥胖的母亲通过改变她们的食品的选择和饮食习惯也可以引起她们子女的饮食习惯的显著的变化（Klohe-Lehman, et al. , 2007）。另一项基于家庭的干预研究也发现，肥胖儿童的 BMI 指数的 Z 分变化受到他们父母的 BMI 指数的 Z 分的影响（Wrotniak, et al. , 2004）。

不过，针对父母的干预方案仍存在一些不足（Golan &

Weizman，2001）。首先，大部分干预方案仍局限于营养问题，身体活动没有得到应有的重视。此外，父母对 12 岁以下的儿童具有很强的影响力。但是，当儿童长大后，他们逐渐变得更独立，他们朋友的影响力则与日俱增（Golan & Weizman，2001）。因此，针对父母的干预方案为儿童肥胖今后的干预和评价提供了理论框架，但仍需要进一步的提高和调整。

# 第九节　总　结

父母在儿童肥胖的发展和预防中的角色是多方面而复杂的。目前关于父母对于儿童肥胖影响的研究显示，父母在儿童肥胖中发挥着非常重要的作用。父母可以通过遗传、父母的认知、父母教养子女的行为、父母教养子女的方式、家庭环境等途径来影响儿童的体重水平。鉴于已经有许多研究证明了父母与儿童肥胖的联系，建议儿童肥胖的干预中应更加重视父母的作用。

# 第三章　调查问卷的信度和效度研究

## 第一节　前　言

青少年时期的肥胖常常会延续到成年时期（Whitaker, et al., 1997），而且青少年肥胖也可能与某些慢性病的发展有关（Gunnell, et al., 1998）。因此，青少年的肥胖问题已经成为了一项受到日趋重视的公共卫生问题。过去 20 年的研究强调了父母的重要性。父母通过他们的教养子女的行为和方式影响着青少年肥胖的发生、发展、预防和治疗（Epstein, et al., 1990；Lindsay, et al., 2006）。

有一些研究在中国人群中调查了父母教养子女的行为、父母教养子女的方式、父母对青少年肥胖程度认知与青少年肥胖的关系，发现了一些非常有趣的研究结果（J. L. Chen & Kennedy, 2004；G. S. Ma, 2005；W. J. Ma, et al., 2001）。比如，有研究发现，民主型教养方式、不良的亲子沟通、糟糕的行为控制可能导致青少年的体重问题（J. L. Chen & Kennedy, 2004）。但是，这些研究一个共同的不足是在这个领域，还没有建立起一套有效、可靠，而且适合测量中国父母教养子女的行为和教养方式的问卷。此外，在许多这类研究中，仅仅测量了一种或两种父母教养子女的行为，而没有全面地测量所有相关的父母教养子女的行为。

虽然有一批具有良好信度、效度的问卷，比如青少年喂养问卷（Child Feeding Questionnaire，CFQ）、家庭饮食和运动习惯问卷（Family Eating and Activity Habits Questionnaire）、监护人喂养方式问卷（Caregiver's Feeding Styles Questionnaire）已经在西方国家编订和使用，但是这些问卷并不能不经过信效度测试而直接用于中国人群。

因此，本次研究的目的是修订和验证适合中国人群的父母教养子女的行为、教养子女的方式和对青少年肥胖程度的认知问卷。

# 第二节　研究方法

## 一、问卷选择

在查阅大量相关文献资料的基础上（Golan & Weizman，2001；Hughes，et al.，2008；Lindsay，et al.，2006；Rhee，2008；Trost，et al.，2003），我们明确了本研究问卷的理论框架，总结了目前现有的各类相关问卷的优点和缺点。因为目前已有几十种问卷用于测量父母教养子女的行为、教养方式和对青少年肥胖程度的认知，因此我们问卷选择采用了以下三个标准：1. 已有研究证明该问卷具有可接受的信度和效度；2. 问卷的问题适合于 10 – 15 岁的青少年；3. 问题不存在文化冲突。我们选择的问卷具体内容包括：

**青少年对体重水平的认知**

研究采用了 Collins 等人设计的几组绘有男孩、女孩、成年男士、成年女性的图画用以测量青少年对他们自身以及他们父母体重水平的认知（Collins，1991）。每组图片包括七个由瘦到胖的青少年（或成人）。青少年会被要求从图中选择他们认为最像自己和最希望的一幅图。这批图片本来是为儿童设计的，但是有研究证实这些图片可以应用于 10 岁以上青少年（Parkinson，et al.，1998）。以一年级到三年级学生为研究对象的测试的 3 天间隔时间的重测信度为 0. 71（Collins，1991）。

**父母对子女体重水平的认知**

为了测量父母对子女体重水平的认知，一个前人研究中使用的题目被用在本研究中（Shi，et al.，2007）。父母们会被要求从 5 个选项中选择一个与他们认为看法最接近的。5 个选项分别是："很瘦"、"有点瘦"、"正常体重"、"有点超重"、"严重超重"。

**父母教养子女的行为**

本研究在前人研究所采用问卷中用于测量父母教养子女的行为的题目（Arredondo，et al.，2006；O'Connor，et al.，2010）的基础上，进行了改编和修订，形成了本次调查的问卷。问卷主要包括："饮食和身体活动的监管"，"把食物或静坐少动行为当作奖励"，"鼓励或强迫子女饮食"，"限制不健康饮食和静坐少动行为"和"对子女饮食和身体活动的鼓励"。研究问卷的问题选项采用李克特五分量表，回答选项包括：“从未”、“很少”、“有时”、“经常”、“总是”，或“完全不同意”、“不同意”、“中立”、“同意”、“完全同意”。

### 父母教养子女的方式

由于只有父母教养子女的方式被青少年感受到才能发挥其应有的作用（Choquet, et al., 2008），因此本研究选择测量的是子女感受到的父母教养子女的方式而不是父母自我报告的教养方式。研究采用的是民主父母教养指数（Authoritative Parenting Index, API）作为测量工具。有研究已经证实了 API 问卷的结构与理论模型相符，且具有良好的重测信度（Jackson, et al., 1998）。API 问卷可以用于小学四年级（9 – 10 岁）到高中一年级（15 – 16 岁）的青少年（Jackson, et al., 1998）。问卷共有16 个题目，其中 9 个题目测量关爱（responsiveness），7 个题目则用于测量控制（demandingness）。

## 二、翻译和回译

本研究的问卷中的题目是来自欧美国家的问卷，需要进行翻译和回译。翻译和回译的步骤是严格遵循跨文化翻译所要求的程序进行的（Banville, et al., 2000）。首先，由两名熟练掌握中英文的研究生将英文的问卷题目翻译成中文。两名研究生完成翻译后，将翻译结果进行对照，讨论两份翻译问卷的不同之处，并最终达成一致的翻译卷。第二，请另外两名熟练掌握中英文的研究生将翻译卷再翻译回英文，两名学生在翻译前并没有看过原英文问卷。对比两名研究生的分别回译问卷，并最终达成一致的回译问卷。第三，将回译问卷与原版英文问卷进行比较，分析存在差异的原因，解决翻译中存在的问题，最终形成翻译问卷。

## 三、内容效度

根据父母教养子女的行为和教养方式的理论框架，研究准备了相关的问卷问题。5 名分别从事家庭研究、营养学、运动科学、体育和医学的专家被邀请评价问卷问题。专家们被告知了问卷的目的，并被要求分别填写一份针对问卷的评价表。他们需要对问卷中的每个问题的有效性进行评价，并可以增加任何他们认为需要的内容。假如问卷的某个问题未得到80%的认可（即5个专家中的4个认为可以保留该问题），则该问题会被删除。问卷的内容通过专家们的评阅得以修改。

## 四、实验版问卷的预实验

在赣州和汕头邀请15 对青少年和父母（7 对来自赣州，8 对来自汕头）参加实验版问卷的测试，并接受访谈。根据 Banville 等人（2000）的推荐，首先邀请青少年及其父母填写实验版问卷，然后请受试对象谈谈问卷内容是否有不能理解的问题或者有令人不悦的问题。此外，受试对象还被邀请谈谈父母教养子女的行为和教养方式，以确定问卷问题是否已经涵盖了父母教养子女的行为和教养方式的主要内容。根据受试对象的反馈，修改问卷的内容和语言，让问卷更符合中国人的实际情况。

## 五、重测信度和内部一致性

有研究推荐进行问卷信度研究需要至少 50 名的受试对象（Hopkins，2000），因此，本问卷共招募了 127 对青少年及其父母作为研究对象（赣州 62 对，汕头 65 对）。在此项信度研究中，青少年和他们的父母需要做两次问卷，两次相隔的时间为两个星期。以这批数据为基础，研究确定问卷的重测信度和内部一致性。

## 六、结构效度

共有 2162 名来自赣州和汕头的青少年及其父母参加了本次调查。从中随机抽取了 1000 个数据用以计算问卷的结构效度。

## 七、数据分析

计算每个问题的组内相关系数（intraclass correlation coefficient，ICC）以确定重测信度。若 ICC 大于 0.7 则该题目的重测信度被接受。计算克隆巴赫系数（Cronbach's alpha）以确定一组亚量表的内部一致性。如果克隆巴赫系数大于 0.6，则认为内部一致性可接受（Sim & Wright，2000）。采用 Lisrel 8.51 软件进行验证性因子分析（Confirmatory Factor Analysis，CFA）确定问卷的结构效度。如果 NNFI（Non-Normed Fit Index）高于 0.90，CFI（Comparative Fit Index）高于 0.90，RMSEA（Root Mean Square Error of Approximation）低于 0.08，则认为问卷的结构符合理论模型（Hooper，et al.，2008）。

# 第三节 结 果

## 一、内容效度

研究分别为青少年和父母的问卷准备了 46 个和 41 个问题。青少年问卷有 6 个问题，父母问卷有 3 个问题未得到 80% 专家的认可，因此被删除。因此，经过内容效度测试，青少年问卷和父母问卷分别有 40 个问题和 38 个问题得到保留。

## 二、重测信度和内部一致性

表 3.1 总结了参加信度测试的受试对象的基本情况。在 127 名青少年中，65 名（51.2%）为男生，60 名（48.8%）为女生。受试青少年的年龄范围为 10 岁到 15 岁。在 127 名受访青少年父母中，80 名为母亲，占总数的 63%。

表 3.1　受试者基本情况（N = 127）

| | |
|---|---|
| 青少年性别，% | |
| 　男生 | 51.2 |
| 　女生 | 48.8 |
| 年龄，平均值 ± 标准差，岁 | 13.1 ± 0.8 |
| 身高，cm | 162.2 ± 6.7 |
| 体重，kg | 50.2 ± 7.6 |
| BMI | 19.1 ± 2.4 |
| 超重，% | 18.1 |
| 父母性别，% | |
| 　男性 | 37.0 |
| 　女性 | 63.0 |

如表 3.2 所示，青少年对体重水平的认知和父母对子女体重水平的认知相关问题的重测信度非常不错，组内相关系数的范围

为 0.82 到 0.92。研究结果显示，青少年对自身体重水平的认知和父母对子女体重水平的认知的相关问题具有良好的可靠性。

**表 3.2  青少年对体重水平的认知和父母对子女体重水平的**

**认知相关问题的重测信度**

| 题目 | ICC | 95% CI | N | P | 报告对象 |
|---|---|---|---|---|---|
| 请选择以下哪幅图最像你？ | 0.92 | 0.89 - 0.95 | 123 | 0.000 | A |
| 请选择下面哪幅图是你希望自己的样子？ | 0.86 | 0.80 - 0.90 | 123 | 0.000 | A |
| 请选择下面哪幅图最像你爸爸的外形？ | 0.91 | 0.87 - 0.94 | 123 | 0.000 | A |
| 请选择下面哪幅图最像你妈妈的外形？ | 0.91 | 0.87 - 0.94 | 123 | 0.000 | A |
| 请选择下面哪幅图是你希望自己长大后的样子？ | 0.83 | 0.76 - 0.88 | 123 | 0.000 | A |
| 请报告你孩子的肥胖程度 | 0.88 | 0.82 - 0.92 | 126 | 0.000 | P |

注：A：青少年  P：父母

如表 3.3 所示，调查父母教养子女的行为题目的重测信度，有一个问题的重测信度低于 0.7，因而该题被删徐。研究结果显示，调查父母教养子女的行为其他题目的重测信度范围是 0.71 到 0.83，内部一致性的范围为 0.69 到 0.79。这一结果表明，问卷题目具有良好的可靠性和内部一致性。

**表 3.3  关于父母教养子女的行为问卷题目的重测信度和内部一致性**

| 问题 | ICC | 95% CI | N | P | 克隆巴赫系数 |
|---|---|---|---|---|---|
| **饮食和身体活动的监管** | | | | | 0.76 |
| 1. 我会关注我的孩子吃甜食的数量（如蛋糕、糖果、冰淇淋） | 0.74 | 0.61 - 0.82 | 125 | .000 | |

| 问题 | ICC | 95% CI | N | P | 克隆巴赫系数 |
|---|---|---|---|---|---|
| 2. 我会关注我的孩子吃高脂食品的数量（如：油炸、膨化食品） | 0.71 | 0.57 – 0.80 | 125 | .000 | |
| 3. 我会关注我的孩子吃蔬菜水果的数量 | 0.80 | 0.70 – 0.86 | 125 | .000 | |
| 4. 我的孩子吃零食之前要经过我同意 | 0.71 | 0.56 – 0.80 | 125 | .000 | |
| 5. 我会关注我的孩子看电视、玩电子游戏、上网的时间 | 0.72 | 0.59 – 0.81 | 125 | .000 | |
| 6. 我会关注我的孩子的体育锻炼的运动强度和时间 | 0.73 | 0.60 – 0.81 | 125 | .000 | |
| **对子女健康饮食和身体活动的鼓励** | | | | | 0.79 |
| 7. 假如我的孩子选择吃健康的食品，我会表扬他/她 | 0.83 | 0.75 – 0.89 | 123 | .000 | |
| 8. 假如我的孩子积极参加体育运动，我会表扬他/她 | 0.71 | 0.57 – 0.81 | 122 | .000 | |
| **把食物或静坐少动行为当作奖励** | | | | | 0.69 |
| 9. 假如孩子表现好，我会给些零食（糖果，冰淇淋等）奖励他/她 | 0.77 | 0.66 – 0.84 | 125 | .000 | |
| 10. 假如孩子表现好，我会让他/她看电视或者玩电子游戏作为奖励 | 0.72 | 0.60 – 0.81 | 125 | .000 | |
| **鼓励或强迫子女饮食** | | | | | 0.74 |
| 11. 我不允许孩子剩饭 | 0.55 | 0.34 – 0.70 | 126 | .000 | D |
| 12. 我应该特别关注，确保让我的孩子吃饱饭 | 0.76 | 0.65 – 0.84 | 126 | .000 | |
| 13. 假如我的孩子说"我吃饱了"，我还是会尽量让他再吃一些 | 0.78 | 0.67 – 0.85 | 124 | .000 | |
| 14. 假如我不对我孩子的饮食加以指导和调节，他就会吃得比他该吃的量少 | 0.71 | 0.56 – 0.80 | 124 | .000 | |

| 问题 | ICC | 95% CI | N | P | 克隆巴赫系数 |
|---|---|---|---|---|---|
| **限制不健康饮食和静坐少动行为** | | | | | 0.74 |
| 15. 我会控制我的孩子喝含糖饮料的量（可乐、雪碧、鲜橙多等） | 0.71 | 0.57 – 0.81 | 124 | .000 | |
| 16. 我会控制我的孩子吃零食的数量 | 0.71 | 0.57 – 0.80 | 124 | .000 | |
| 17. 周一到周五，我会控制孩子看电视、玩电子游戏的时间 | 0.81 | 0.73 – 0.87 | 124 | .000 | |
| 18. 周末，我会控制孩子看电视、玩电子游戏的时间 | 0.83 | 0.75 – 0.89 | 124 | .000 | |

注：D：该项问题被删除，克隆巴赫系数的计算是基于重测信度高于 0.7 的题目。

本次研究的结果还显示，测量父母教养子女的方式的问题也具有较好的重测信度和内部一致性。如表 3.4 和 3.5 所示，母亲 16 个题目的重测信度的范围为 0.70 – 0.84，父亲为 0.70 – 0.85。父亲和母亲在关爱和控制两个亚量表的内部一致性为 0.70 到 0.75。这些结果表明，问卷具有较好的可靠性。

**表 3.4 关于父亲教养方式问卷题目的重测信度和内部一致性**

| 问题 | ICC | 95% CI | N | P | 克隆巴赫系数 |
|---|---|---|---|---|---|
| **关爱（父亲）** | | | | | 0.70 |
| 1. 我爸爸不让我自己决定事情该怎么做，总是吩咐我该怎么做 | 0.72 | 0.60 – 0.80 | 123 | .000 | |
| 2. 我爸爸制定规矩（如：我可以几点钟出去玩）从来不考虑我的想法 | 0.75 | 0.64 – 0.82 | 123 | .000 | |
| 3. 当我心情不好时，我爸爸总能让我感觉好起来 | 0.71 | 0.59 – 0.80 | 123 | .000 | |

| 问题 | ICC | 95% CI | N | P | 克隆巴赫系数 |
|---|---|---|---|---|---|
| 4. 我爸爸总是太忙，都没有空跟我聊聊天 | 0.75 | 0.64 – 0.82 | 123 | .000 | |
| 5. 我爸爸总会倾听我说的话 | 0.73 | 0.62 – 0.81 | 123 | .000 | |
| 6. 在我爸爸面前，我可以说真心话，表现真实的自己，不需要任何遮掩 | 0.71 | 0.57 – 0.79 | 123 | .000 | |
| 7. 当我表现好的时候，我爸爸会表扬我 | 0.78 | 0.69 – 0.85 | 123 | .000 | |
| 8. 我爸爸愿意听我说我遇到的困难 | 0.76 | 0.65 – 0.83 | 123 | .000 | |
| 9. 我的表现无论好坏，我爸爸都喜欢 | 0.82 | 0.74 – 0.87 | 123 | .000 | |
| 控制（父亲） | | | | | 0.75 |
| 10. 我爸爸制定的规矩（如：我可以几点钟出去玩），我必须遵守 | 0.72 | 0.60 – 0.81 | 123 | .000 | |
| 11. 我爸爸会叮嘱我必须几点几点前回家 | 0.72 | 0.60 – 0.81 | 123 | .000 | |
| 12. 我去什么地方必须得告诉我爸爸 | 0.71 | 0.59 – 0.80 | 123 | .000 | |
| 13. 我爸爸总是让我准时睡觉 | 0.75 | 0.64 – 0.82 | 123 | .000 | |
| 14. 我爸爸会过问我和朋友们都干了些什么 | 0.70 | 0.57 – 0.79 | 123 | .000 | |
| 15. 我爸爸清楚我放学以后去什么地方 | 0.85 | 0.78 – 0.89 | 123 | .000 | |
| 16. 我爸爸会检查我是否做完我的家庭作业 | 0.75 | 0.64 – 0.83 | 123 | .000 | |

注：D：该项问题被删除，克隆巴赫系数的计算是基于重测信度高于 0.7 的题目。

表 3.5　关于母亲教养方式问卷题目的重测信度和内部一致性

| 问题 | ICC | 95% CI | N | P | 克隆巴赫系数 |
|---|---|---|---|---|---|
| **关爱（母亲）** | | | | | 0.71 |
| 1. 我妈妈不让我自己决定事情该怎么做，总是吩咐我该怎么做 | 0.74 | 0.62－0.82 | 122 | .000 | |
| 2. 我妈妈制定规矩（如：我可以几点钟出去玩）从来不考虑我的想法 | 0.75 | 0.65－0.83 | 123 | .000 | |
| 3. 当我心情不好时，我妈妈总能让我感觉好起来 | 0.72 | 0.59－0.80 | 123 | .000 | |
| 4. 我妈妈总是太忙，都没有空跟我聊聊天 | 0.70 | 0.58－0.79 | 123 | .000 | |
| 5. 我妈妈总会倾听我说的话 | 0.73 | 0.61－0.81 | 123 | .000 | |
| 6. 在我妈妈面前，我可以说真心话，表现真实的自己，不需要任何遮掩 | 0.70 | 0.57－0.79 | 123 | .000 | |
| 7. 当我表现好的时候，我妈妈会表扬我 | 0.84 | 0.76－0.89 | 123 | .000 | |
| 8. 我妈妈愿意听我说我遇到的困难 | 0.76 | 0.65－0.83 | 123 | .000 | |
| 9. 我的表现无论好坏，我妈妈都喜欢 | 0.73 | 0.61－0.81 | 122 | .000 | |
| **控制（母亲）** | | | | | 0.71 |
| 10. 我妈妈制定的规矩（如：我可以几点钟出去玩），我必须遵守 | 0.74 | 0.63－0.82 | 123 | .000 | |
| 11. 我妈妈会叮嘱我必须几点几点前回家 | 0.70 | 0.56－0.79 | 123 | .000 | |

| 问题 | ICC | 95% CI | N | P | 克隆巴赫系数 |
|---|---|---|---|---|---|
| 12. 我去什么地方必须得告诉我妈妈 | 0.74 | 0.63 – 0.82 | 123 | .000 | |
| 13. 我妈妈总是让我准时睡觉 | 0.72 | 0.59 – 0.80 | 123 | .000 | |
| 14. 我妈妈会过问我和朋友们都干了些什么 | 0.75 | 0.64 – 0.82 | 123 | .000 | |
| 15. 我妈妈清楚我放学以后去什么地方 | 0.74 | 0.62 – 0.82 | 123 | .000 | |
| 16. 我妈妈会检查我是否做完我的家庭作业 | 0.70 | 0.58 – 0.79 | 123 | .000 | |

注：D：该项问题被删除，克隆巴赫系数的计算是基于重测信度高于 0.7 的题目。

经过信度测试，仅有一个父母问卷的题目被删除，青少年问卷还有 40 个题目，而父母问卷还有 38 个题目。

## 三、结构效度

如表 3.6 所示，验证性因子分析的结果显示，父母教养子女的行为各因子载荷的范围为 0.60 到 0.76。从验证性因子分析的拟合指数来看（RMSEA = 0.052，NNFI = 0.91，CFI = 0.92），模型拟合效果较好。表 3.7 总结了父母教养子女的方式问卷的验证性因子分析结果，父亲和母亲问卷中各因子载荷结果相似，父亲卷因子载荷的范围为 0.55 到 0.76，母亲卷因子载荷为 0.59 到 0.74。RMSEA、CFI、NNFI 等拟合指数的结果也显示，问卷结构符合理论框架。

### 表 3.6　父母教养子女的行为问卷中各问题的因子载荷

| 题目 | 因子载荷[a] |
|---|---|
| **饮食和身体活动的监管** | |
| 1. 我会关注我的孩子吃甜食的数量（如蛋糕、糖果、冰淇淋） | 0.67 |
| 2. 我会关注我的孩子吃高脂食品的数量（如：油炸、膨化食品） | 0.68 |
| 3. 我会关注我的孩子吃蔬菜水果的数量 | 0.66 |
| 4. 我的孩子吃零食之前要经过我同意 | 0.72 |
| 5. 我会关注我的孩子看电视、玩电子游戏、上网的时间 | 0.69 |
| 6. 我会关注我的孩子的体育锻炼的运动强度和时间 | 0.74 |
| **对子女健康饮食和身体活动的鼓励** | |
| 7. 假如我的孩子选择吃健康的食品，我会表扬他/她 | 0.65 |
| 8. 假如我的孩子积极参加体育运动，我会表扬他/她 | 0.70 |
| **把食物或静坐少动行为当作奖励** | |
| 9. 假如孩子表现好，我会给些零食（糖果，冰淇淋等）奖励他/她 | 0.76 |
| 10. 假如孩子表现好，我会让他/她看电视或者玩电子游戏作为奖励 | 0.65 |
| **鼓励或强迫子女饮食** | |
| 11. 我应该特别关注，确保让我的孩子吃饱饭 | 0.71 |
| 12. 假如我的孩子说"我吃饱了"，我还是会尽量让他再吃一些 | 0.70 |
| 13. 假如我不对我孩子的饮食加以指导和调节，他就会吃得比他该吃的量少 | 0.68 |
| **限制不健康饮食和静坐少动行为** | |
| 14. 我会控制我的孩子喝含糖饮料的量（可乐、雪碧、鲜橙多等） | 0.60 |
| 15. 我会控制我的孩子吃零食的数量 | 0.74 |
| 16. 周一到周五，我会控制孩子看电视、玩电子游戏的时间 | 0.74 |
| 17. 周末，我会控制孩子看电视、玩电子游戏的时间 | 0.71 |

[a] 验证性因子分析拟合指数情况：RMSEA = 0.052，NNFI = 0.91，CFI = 0.92。

表 3.7　父母教养子女的方式问卷中各问题的因子载荷

| 题目 | 因子载荷 | |
| --- | --- | --- |
| | 父亲卷 | 母亲卷 |
| **关爱** | | |
| 1. 我爸爸/妈妈不让我自己决定事情该怎么做，总是吩咐我该怎么做 | 0.64 | 0.65 |
| 2. 我爸爸/妈妈制定规矩（如：我可以几点钟出去玩）从来不考虑我的想法 | 0.64 | 0.66 |
| 3. 当我心情不好时，我爸爸/妈妈总能让我感觉好起来 | 0.69 | 0.67 |
| 4. 我爸爸/妈妈总是太忙，都没有空跟我聊聊天 | 0.62 | 0.61 |
| 5. 我爸爸/妈妈总会倾听我说的话. | 0.68 | 0.66 |
| 6. 在我爸爸/妈妈面前，我可以说真心话，表现真实的自己，不需要任何遮掩。 | 0.65 | 0.69 |
| 7. 当我表现好的时候，我爸爸/妈妈会表扬我 | 0.62 | 0.61 |
| 8. 我爸爸/妈妈愿意听我说我遇到的困难。 | 0.55 | 0.59 |
| 9. 我的表现无论好坏，我爸爸/妈妈都喜欢。 | 0.63 | 0.63 |
| **控制（父亲）** | | |
| 10. 我爸爸/妈妈制定的规矩（如：我可以几点钟出去玩），我必须遵守 | 0.70 | 0.69 |
| 11. 我爸爸/妈妈会叮嘱我必须几点几点前回家 | 0.62 | 0.66 |
| 12. 我去什么地方必须得告诉我爸爸/妈妈 | 0.72 | 0.73 |
| 13. 我爸爸/妈妈总是让我准时睡觉 | 0.66 | 0.64 |
| 14. 我爸爸/妈妈会过问我和朋友们都干了些什么 | 0.76 | 0.74 |
| 15. 我爸爸/妈妈清楚我放学以后去什么地方 | 0.68 | 0.68 |
| 16. 我爸爸/妈妈会检查我是否做完我的家庭作业 | 0.65 | 0.67 |

验证性因子分析拟合指数情况：父亲卷 RMSEA = 0.056，NNFI = 0.92，CFI = 0.93；母亲卷：RMSEA = 0.055，NNFI = 0.93，CFI = 0.94。

# 第四节　讨论与结论

本项研究的目的确定用以测量父母教养子女的行为、父母教养子女的方式以及父母对子女体重水平认知问卷的效度和信度。此项研究验证了问卷的内容效度、结构效度、两周重测信度和内部一致性。研究数据显示问卷的效度和信度均处于可接受范围内，可以用于中国青少年及其父母。

前期的研究发现，父母的一些行为可能与青少年肥胖有关。比如，近年来的研究指出，父母喂养子女或为子女提供食物这一行为对青少年食物摄入具有重要影响（Koletzko, et al., 2009; Kroller & Warschburger, 2009）。在前人研究的理论框架和问卷的基础上（Arredondo, et al., 2006; O'Connor, et al., 2010），本研究修订了有 17 个题目的父母教养子女的行为问卷。问卷主要包括了"饮食和身体活动的监管"，"把食物或静坐少动行为当作奖励"，"鼓励或强迫子女饮食"，"限制不健康饮食和静坐少动行为"和"对子女饮食和身体活动的鼓励"五个维度，这五个维度也是前期研究中发现影响青少年肥胖的发展的重要因素（Clark, et al., 2007; Faith, Scanlon, et al., 2004; Rhee, 2008）。验证性因子分析的拟合指数显示，问卷的结构符合理论模型。问卷的内容效度、两周重测信度和内部一致性均在可接受范围内。

在本研究中，用以测量父母教养子女的方式的题目，来源于民主父母教养指数（Authoritative Parenting Index, API）。已经有研究证明了 API 问卷的效度和信度。父母教养子女的方式有关爱和控制两个维度，而前期的研究也证明了该问卷的结构符合这一理论模型（Jackson, et al. , 1998）。本研究则进一步验证了该问卷的有效性和可靠性。但是，也必须考虑到中西方国家在父母教养子女的方式上可能存在差异。比如，欧美人比较重视培养和保护青少年先天的个性和能力。但是，中国人比较强调自律、尊重父母、父母的作用，这些都是植根于我国的儒家教育思想（Chao, 1994; F. M. Chen & Luster, 2002）。因此，有中国学者认为民主和专制这些父母教养子女的方式并没有完全体现中国父母教养子女方式的特点（Chao, 1994）。此外，目前对于父母教养子女方式的评价和分类并没有一个"临界值"。父母教养子女方式的分类是采用研究群体在关爱和控制两个维度得分的中位数将受试对象分为四类（Darling & Steinberg, 1993）。因此，父母教养子女方式的界定是基于一种相对，而不是绝对的方法进行。考虑到中美父母在教养子女方式上可能存在的差异（P. Wu, et al. , 2002），一个中国研究中的放任型父母假如放在一个美国的研究中可能成为一名民主型父母。因此，对于父母教养子女方式的测量问题还需要进一步的研究。

需要指出的是，本研究仍存在一些不足。首先，目前还没有一套成熟的中国父母教养子女方式的理论，虽然本研究中在问卷编订过程中也尽量去处理了中西方文化差异问题，但是本研究的问卷还是建立在西方国家相应的父母教养子女方式理论的基础上。因此，问卷可能存在没有完全涵盖中国父母教养子女方式和行为的特点。不过需要指出的是，尽管如此，这一来自西方的父母教养子女方式理论（Baumrind，1971）已经广泛应用于中国的父母教养子女方式的研究中（X. Y. Chen，et al.，1997；Pong，et al.，2009；Porter，et al.，2005），并取得了不错的研究成果，这也证明该理论仍能够帮助我们解决中国的相关研究问题。因此，本研究问卷，仍然对于我国后续的父母教养子女的方式研究具有重要意义。第二，在重测信度的测试上，记忆问题是难以避免的。虽然研究间隔了两周，但是青少年和父母们在进行第二次问卷测试时，可能仍记得他们第一次测试时选择的答案。因而，这一问题也可能导致重测信度被高估。第三，虽然我们要求进行重测信度的两次测试，青少年应尽量找同一名家长填写问卷，即第一次测试为父亲填写，第二次测试仍应找父亲填写问卷。但是，也不排除有部分受试者未严格遵守研究要求，这也可能导致问卷的重测信度被低估。此外，本次研究的对象为赣州市和汕头市 10 – 15 岁青少年及其父母。因此，研究制订的问卷可能并不适用于 10 岁以下儿童及其家长。问卷是否适用于我国其他地区也需要进一步的验证。

综上所述，本研究为制订的问卷提供了内容效度、结构效度、重测信度和内部一致性的相关数据。虽然研究仍存在一些不足，但是研究也能够证明该青少年问卷和父母问卷具有良好的信度和效度，可以应月于我国青少年和父母人群，用以测量父母对子女体重的认知、父母教养子女的行为和教养方式。

# 第四章 父母教养子女的行为与青少年肥胖

## 第一节 前 言

虽然在一些发展中国家青少年的营养不良问题依然严峻，但是目前的研究发现，在许多发展中国家，特别是一些经济高速发展的国家，年轻女性超重的比例高于低体重的比例（Mendez, et al., 2005）。比如，最近在我国的研究发现，青少年群体体重指数（BMI）的第 95 百分位数增长非常迅速（Popkin, 2010）。这预示着，中国的儿童肥胖问题可能会像美国一样成为日益严重的公共卫生问题。

专家们推荐采用均衡的饮食、增加身体活动量和增加社会支持等办法来改变人们饮食和生活习惯，从而解决肥胖问题（Heber, 2010）。还有学者强调了父母的参与在青少年体重控制当中的作用（Barlow & the Expert Committee, 2007）。有一些学者建议对于青少年肥胖的干预必须有至少一名家长参与（Dietz & Robinson, 2005；Robinson, 1999）。近年来，质化研究和量化研究的研究结果都表明父母的参与对于青少年肥胖的干预非常重要（Heinberg, et al., 2009；Stewart, et al., 2008）。

父母不仅通过他们提供的家庭环境、他们在抚养子女中的饮食方法（禁止子女吃某些食品，鼓励子女吃某些食品，把食物当作子女表现好的奖励等）、他们在经济上和感情上的支持，影响着他们子女的饮食和身体活动，还通过他们自身的"榜样作用"影响着子女饮食和锻炼习惯的养成。比如，有一项纵向跟踪研究发现，在控制了先天因素（青少年3岁时的体重指数）影响的基础上，假如家长们在子女5岁时禁止子女吃某些食品，可能导致他们在7岁时体重指数更高（Faith, Berkowitz, et al., 2004）。有研究人员解释，这可能是因为父母禁止青少年吃某些食品，反而引起了青少年对受禁食品的注意和食欲（Fisher & Birch, 1999b）。Framingham青少年研究的结果则发现，经常积极参与身体活动的父母，其子女积极参与身体活动的比例也高于身体活动不积极父母的子女（Moore, et al., 1991）。

但是，也有一些研究的结果不尽相同。比如，有研究发现，受到父母鼓励的青少年每周积极参与身体活动的天数比那些没有受到父母鼓励的青少年多（King, et al., 2008）。但是，另一项研究却发现，女生身体活动水平与她们感受到的父母对她们参与身体活动的支持不相关（Adkins, et al., 2004）。因此，还需要进一步的研究，以确定父母教养子女的行为是否与青少年的饮食和身体活动有关，这对于青少年肥胖的预防和干预非常重要。

在中国，也有学者研究了中国父母教养子女的行为与青少年肥胖的关系。比如，一项调查了北京 930 户家庭的横向调查发现，父母的饮食习惯、看电视行为以及身体活动量与其子女的饮食习惯、看电视行为和身体活动量高度相关（Jiang, et al., 2006）。另一项来自香港地区 104 名青少年父母的研究发现，父亲的榜样作用显著地影响了超重青少年的身体活动量（Lau, et al., 2007）。但是，这些研究大部分都仅仅关注了一两种父母教养子女的行为，而没有全面研究父母的其他教养行为。另外，我们还需要关注在父母教养子女的行为中的文化因素。比如，在中国文化中，父亲被认为应该是"严"的，而母亲被认为应该是"慈"的。因此，中国父亲和母亲在家庭中扮演的角色是不同的，因而教养子女的行为也可能有所区别。但是，很少有研究比较中国父亲和母亲在饮食和身体活动相关的教养子女行为上有何差异。

因此，本次研究的目的有：1. 研究青少年的饮食习惯、身体活动水平、体重水平与其父母教养子女的行为的关系；2. 比较中国父亲和母亲在饮食和身体活动相关的教养行为上有何差异。

## 第二节　研究方法

### 研究对象与方案

本文调查对象选取了中国南方的两个城市的青少年及其父母，因为与农村地区相比，城市地区的肥胖问题更严重（Luo & Hu, 2002）。由于经济和社会发展与人们的高热量食物摄入、静坐少动行为、肥胖超重问题有关（Y. Wang, et al. , 2002），因此本研究决定在我国南方的发达地区和欠发达地区分别抽取研究对象。研究采用随机分层抽样法，抽取汕头市作为南方发达地区代表，赣州市作为南方欠发达地区代表。汕头是我国 20 世纪 80 年代最早建立的经济特区之一。根据 2010 年汕头市政府统计公报的数据，汕头市 2010 年人均 GDP 为 20279 元（Shantou municipal bureau of statistics, 2010）。赣州作为我国的革命老区，是一个欠发达的内陆城市。根据 2010 年赣州市政府统计公报的数据，赣州市人 2010 年人均 GDP 为 9391 元。

研究随机选取这两个城市初中一年级和二年级的青少年及其父母作为调查对象。以赣州为例，赣州有两个行政区。在本研究中，在每个区抽取一所重点中学和一所普通中学，每所中学抽取 4 - 6 个班级（每个年级 2 - 3 个班）。同样的抽样策略也应用于汕头市。青少年如果曾接受过可能影响其体重的治疗，或者存在身体残疾或慢性病，不能作为本研究的研究对象。

在 2009 年 4 月到 5 月，有 2162 组青少年及其父母参与了本次调查（其中赣州 1179 组，汕头 1106 组），其中 19 位青少年由于存在身体残疾或需要接受药物治疗会影响其体重，所以不将其纳入研究分析。在调查过程中，274 位家长未交回调查问卷，最终有 2143 位青少年以及 1869 位家长的调查数据被纳入数据分析。

在调查中，青少年们需要完成身高与体重的测量，然后在教室填写一份问卷，如有需要，调查人员将提供帮助。然后青少年要将新的问卷带回家让其父母填写（父亲或母亲都可以填写问卷）。随后问卷将统一由调查人员收集，调查人员会向被调查者送上小礼物以示感谢。

另有 127 组青少年及其父母（赣州 62 组，汕头 65 组）在开展调查前四周对问卷进行可靠性检验，相隔两周重复完成这份问卷。问卷的再测信度和内在一致性通过同类相关系数和克隆巴赫系数分别进行验证。

在调查之前需要获得调查对象的署名同意。父母被引导提供关于其子女健康状况的信息并鼓励青少年及父母按真实想法作答。在问卷调查中答案不分对错，而且调查人员将对问卷严格保密。研究获得了香港中文大学研究伦理委员会的正式许可。

**主要调查指标**

**青少年体重水平**

对青少年体重的测量精确到 0.1 千克（脱鞋、穿尽量少的衣服），身高测量精确到 0.5 厘米。并计算出体重指数（BMI），计算公式为 BMI = 体重（kg）/身高（m）$^2$，其标准定为偏瘦（调整年龄性别后的体重水平低于平均体重 2 个标准差）、正常或超重（调整年龄性别后的体重水平高于平均体重 1 个标准差），该标准是世界健康组织（WHO）根据世界青少年（学生时期青少年）成长标准制定的（Butte, et al., 2007; De Onis, et al., 2007）。根据国际儿童发育标准，计算调整年龄性别后的 BMI 指数的 Z 分（Z – BMI）。

**父母体重水平**

由于测量父母身高体重的可行性不高，因此父母的 BMI 指数是通过其问卷中的身高、体重计算得出。问卷中填写的身高体重的有效性度已经得到了验证（Bolton-Smith, et al., 2000;

Wada, et al., 2005）。调查对象的问卷 BMI 值与实测值的皮尔森相关系数分别为男性 0.943 和女性 0.950 （Wada et al. 2005）。根据超重和肥胖的 BMI 诊断标准，成人的 BMI 值标准为不超重（BMI < 24kg/m$^2$），超重（24kg/m2 ≤ BMI < 28kg/m$^2$），肥胖（BMI≥28kg/m$^2$）（Zhou & Cooperative Meta-Analysis Group of the Working Group on Obesity in China, 2002）。

### 青少年的饮食习惯

采用 12 项的李克特五点量表测量青少年的饮食习惯。在调查中，青少年通过五个回答选项（"从不"、"很少"、"有时"、"经常"和"总是"）来回答关于他们饮食行为习惯的问题。问题例子："我每天吃至少三份水果"、"假如饭菜味道好，我会多吃一点"。有研究显示该问卷具有良好的可靠性和有效性（Sheu, 2003）。本研究的可靠性测试显示，该问卷题目的两周重复性信度为 0.70 - 0.79，问卷的内部一致性为 0.71。

### 青少年的身体活动水平

受试青少年被邀请填写儿童青少年身体活动水平问卷（PARCY）以评价他们过去一年的每周平均活动水平。PARCY 是在 Jackson Activity Coding 问卷（Baumgartner & Jackson, 1996; George, et al., 1997）和 Godin-Shephard Activity Questionnaire 问卷（Aaron, et al., 1993; Godin & Shephard, 1985）的基础上改编的单问题量表。PARCY 问卷的效标效度和同证效度也已经被其他一些研究所证实（Hui, 2001; Hui, et al., 2001; Kong, et al., 2010）。PARCY 问卷是一个 11 分（0 - 10 级）的量表，0 级为完全没有任何身体活动，而 10 级为每天都有大量剧烈身体

活动。受试者们的身体活动水平可以进一步分为"身体活动不足"（PARCY = 0 to 2）、身体活动量中等（PARCY =3 to 6）、身体活动量充足（PARCY = 7 to 10）。本次研究的可靠性测试显示，该量表的两周重测信度为0.83。

**父母教养子女的行为**

采用17项的李克特五点量表，这一问卷是在原有前人研究基础上进行修改和翻译得出的（Arredondo, et al., 2006; O'Connor, et al., 2010），用于评价父母对子女的教养子女的行为。这一量表包括以下子项目："饮食和身体活动的监管"，"把食物或静坐少动行为当作奖励"，"鼓励或强迫子女饮食"，"限制不健康饮食和静坐少动行为"和"对子女饮食和身体活动的鼓励"。李克特五点量表提供可能的选项分别是：从不、极少、有时、经常、总是或者非常不同意、不同意、不确定、同意、非常同意。父母的教养子女的行为各个子项数据相加得出总分。有遗漏的数据用其他教养子女的行为的平均值代替。在父母教养子女的行为子项中，最高的遗漏数据百分比为0.9%。本研究还随机从大样本中抽取1000名受试者数据对问卷的结构效度进行了验证。本研究选用LISREL 8.51版统计软件进行实证的因子分析，关于该问卷的结构效度和重测信度结果请参考第三章中的表3.3和表3.6。

**青少年发育程度**

虽然有许多研究已经发现青少年的肥胖程度与其发育时间密切相关（Kaplowitz, et al., 2001; Tremblay & Frigon, 2005），但是目前对于青少年肥胖的研究并没有很好地控制青少年发育程度对研究结果的影响（Tsiros, et al., 2008）。在本次研究中，采用了一个自评问卷，请青少年报告他们的阴毛、性器官、乳房（仅针对女生）发育情况，以确定青少年的发育程度。有研究发现该问卷测量青少年发育状况具有良好的可靠性（Chan, et al., 2008）。本研究的前期研究发现，该问卷两个题目的两周重测信度分别为0.80和0.82，内部一致性为0.71。

### 其他信息

从问卷中获得青少年的性别和年龄，其他背景信息，比如父母教育程度、父母年龄以及家庭收入通过父母问卷获得。

### 数理统计

分别计算赣州和汕头青少年BMI、Z-BMI、饮食行为习惯、身体活动水平、父母教养子女的行为、父母教养子女的方式以及其他变量的相关系数。由于年龄、性别、社会经济地位等变量与青少年的体重水平、饮食习惯和身体活动存在相关，因此这些变量将作为数据分析中的控制变量（Y. Wang et al., 2002; Y. Wang & Zhang, 2006）。以各种父母教养子女的行为和其他信息变量作为自变量，采用分层多元回归的方法，分别预测青少年的Z-BMI、饮食习惯和身体活动水平。可能与青少年肥胖、饮食行为和身体活动水平有关的变量（比如：性别、年龄、父母教育程度、家庭收入等）作为回归分析中的控制变量第一批进入回归方程。父母自我报告的教养行为和青少年报告的父母教养子女的行为则作为预测变量第二批进入回归方程。研究还将采用协方差分析，比较父亲和母亲的教养行为，协方差分析将控制青少年体重水平、性别、年龄等变量。

# 第三节　研究结果

受试对象的基本情况如表 4.1 所示。本次研究中青少年的年龄为 10 到 15 岁。研究结果显示有 16.7% 的青少年超重。

**表 4.1　受试对象基本情况 （N = 2143）**

| | |
|---|---|
| 青少年性别，% | |
| 　男生 | 51.4 |
| 　女生 | 48.6 |
| 青少年年龄，平均值 ± 标准差，岁 | 12.5 ± 0.9 |
| 青少年体重水平，% | |
| 　体重偏低 | 2.4 |
| 　正常 | 80.9 |
| 　超重 | 16.7 |
| 青少年 BMI，平均值 ± 标准差 | 18.6 ± 2.8 |
| 青少年饮食习惯，平均值 ± 标准差 | 39.3 ± 5.3 |
| 青少年身体活动水平，平均值 ± 标准差 | 5.1 ± 2.8 |
| 父母性别，% | |
| 　男性 | 40.4 |
| 　女性 | 59.6 |
| 父母 BMI，平均值 ± 标准差 | 22.2 ± 3.0 |
| 父母教养子女的行为，平均值 ± 标准差 | |
| 　饮食和身体活动的监管 | 19.8 ± 4.3 |
| 　把食物或静坐少动行为当作奖励 | 5.4 ± 1.8 |
| 　鼓励或强迫子女饮食 | 9.8 ± 2.1 |
| 　限制不健康饮食和静坐少动行为 | 15.4 ± 2.7 |
| 　对子女健康饮食和身体活动的鼓励 | 7.0 ± 2.1 |
| 地区，% | |
| 　赣州 | 45.7 |
| 　汕头 | 54.3 |

表4.2分别总结了赣州和汕头青少年 BMI、饮食习惯、身体活动水平与父母教养子女的行为、教养子女方式以及父母对子女体重认知等变量协相关系数矩阵，协相关系数控制了年龄、性别、家庭收入和父母教育水平等变量的影响。如表4.2所示，汕头和赣州青少年的 BMI 与父母教养子女的行为"饮食和身体活动的监管"的协相关系数分别为0.10和0.12，且协相关系数具有统计学意义（$p < 0.01$）。而汕头和赣州青少年身体活动水平与父母教养子女的行为"对子女饮食和身体活动的鼓励"的协相关系数分别为0.05和0.02，协相关系数均不具有统计学意义。如表4.2所示，汕头和赣州两地受试者在绝大部分变量间的协相关系数都比较接近，因此在后续的数据分析中，将两地受试对象数据合并计算和分析。

表4.2　赣州和汕头青少年 BMI、饮食习惯、身体活动水平与
父母教养子女的行为、教养方式以及父母对子女
体重认知等变量协相关系数矩阵

| | BMI | | Z–BMI | | 饮食习惯 | | 身体活动 | |
|---|---|---|---|---|---|---|---|---|
| | 汕头 | 赣州 | 汕头 | 赣州 | 汕头 | 赣州 | 汕头 | 赣州 |
| 饮食和身体活动的监管 | 0.10* | 0.12* | 0.09* | 0.10* | 0.21* | 0.23* | 0.11* | 0.15* |
| 对子女健康饮食和身体活动的鼓励 | 0.01 | 0.05 | 0.00 | 0.03 | 0.10* | 0.09* | 0.05 | 0.02 |
| 把食物或静坐少动行为当作奖励 | −0.02 | 0.01 | −0.03 | 0.00 | −0.04 | −0.02 | 0.00 | 0.03 |
| 鼓励或强迫子女饮食 | −0.22* | −0.18* | −0.23* | −0.22* | −0.06 | −0.03 | 0.04 | 0.01 |
| 限制不健康饮食和静坐少动行为 | 0.03 | 0.02 | 0.01 | 0.00 | 0.19* | 0.23* | 0.08* | 0.11* |

| | BMI | | Z – BMI | | 饮食习惯 | | 身体活动 | |
|---|---|---|---|---|---|---|---|---|
| | 汕头 | 赣州 | 汕头 | 赣州 | 汕头 | 赣州 | 汕头 | 赣州 |
| 青少年对自我体重水平的认知 | 0.72* | 0.68* | 0.72* | 0.69* | 0.09* | 0.10* | -0.02 | 0.01 |
| 父母对子女体重水平的认知 | 0.75* | 0.65* | 0.74* | 0.65* | 0.09* | 0.07* | 0.00 | 0.05 |
| 父亲的关爱 | -0.01 | 0.05 | -0.02 | 0.04 | 0.20* | 0.16* | 0.12* | 0.08* |
| 母亲的关爱 | 0.00 | 0.01 | -0.01 | 0.01 | 0.18* | 0.17* | 0.10* | 0.09* |
| 父亲的控制 | -0.03 | 0.02 | -0.03 | 0.02 | 0.11* | 0.08* | 0.10* | 0.08* |
| 母亲的控制 | -0.03 | 0.01 | -0.03 | 0.01 | 0.10* | 0.08* | 0.10* | 0.08* |

备注：协相关系数控制了年龄、性别、家庭收入和父母教育程度；* : $p < 0.01$

表 4.3 总结了与饮食和身体活动相关的父母教养子女的行为。研究结果显示，父亲和母亲在"限制不健康饮食和静坐少动行为"、"鼓励或强迫子女饮食"、"对子女健康饮食和身体活动的鼓励"上的差异不具有统计学意义。父亲和母亲在"饮食和身体活动的监管"和"把食物或静坐少动行为当作奖励"两类教养行为上的差异虽然具有统计学差异，但是差异非常小。

**表 4.3 父亲和母亲教养行为的比较**

| 父母教养子女的行为，平均值（95%置信区间） | 母亲 | 父亲 | ANCOVA | |
|---|---|---|---|---|
| | | | F | P |
| 饮食和身体活动的监管 | 20.5（20.2 – 20.9）** | 19.4（19.0 – 19.9）** | 14.11 | <0.01 |
| 把食物或静坐少动行为当作奖励 | 5.5（5.3 – 5.7）* | 5.3（5.1 – 5.4）* | 4.01 | <0.05 |

| 父母教养子女的行为，平均值（95%置信区间） | 母亲 | 父亲 | ANCOVA | |
|---|---|---|---|---|
| | | | F | P |
| 鼓励或强迫子女饮食 | 8.4（8.3 – 8.6） | 8.3（8.2 – 8.5） | 1.10 | >0.05 |
| 限制不健康饮食和静坐少动行为 | 15.6（15.4 – 15.8） | 15.2（15.5） | 3.45 | >0.05 |
| 对子女健康饮食和身体活动的鼓励 | 7.2（7.0 – 7.3） | 7.1（6.8 – 7.3） | 0.43 | >0.05 |

备注：协方差分析控制了青少年体重水平、性别、年龄、父母体重水平和家庭收入等变量；$^*$：$P < 0.05$；$^{**}$：$P < 0.01$

表4.4总结了，合并两地数据后，青少年体重水平、饮食习惯、身体活动水平和父母教养子女的行为的相关系数。如表4.4所示，研究数据显示，青少年报告的几类父母教养子女的行为，包括"鼓励或强迫子女饮食"、"饮食和身体活动的监管"与青少年的BMI和Z－BMI相关，虽然相关系数不高，但是均具有统计学意义。另外，值得注意的是"鼓励或强迫子女饮食"行为与青少年的BMI呈负相关，这也表明，青少年的BMI越高，父母采用"鼓励或强迫子女饮食"行为的可能性就越低。

此外，"饮食和身体活动的监管"、"对子女健康饮食和身体活动的鼓励"、"限制不健康饮食和静坐少动行为"则被发现与青少年的饮食行为呈正相关。另一方面，"饮食和身体活动的监管"、"对子女健康饮食和身体活动的鼓励"还被发现与青少年的身体活动水平相关，虽然相关系数较低，但仍具有统计学意义。

表4.4  青少年BMI、饮食习惯、身体活动水平与父母教养子女的行为的协相关系数矩阵（两地数据合并后）

| | BMI | Z – BMI | 饮食行为 | 身体活动水平 |
|---|---|---|---|---|
| 饮食和身体活动的监管 | 0.10** | 0.09** | 0.21** | 0.11** |
| 对子女健康饮食和身体活动的鼓励 | 0.01 | 0.00 | 0.10** | 0.05 |
| 把食物或静坐少动行为当作奖励 | – 0.02 | – 0.03 | – 0.04 | 0.00 |
| 鼓励或强迫子女饮食 | – 0.22** | – 0.23** | – 0.06 | 0.04 |
| 限制不健康饮食和静坐少动行为 | 0.03 | 0.01 | 0.19** | 0.08* |

备注：协相关系数控制了年龄、性别、家庭收入和父母教育程度；$*$: $p < 0.05$；$**$: $p < 0.01$

研究采用分层多元回归的方法，建立预测青少年 Z – BMI、饮食习惯和身体活动水平的预测方程。如表4.5所示，回归模型控制了一些受试者的基本信息变量，如性别、年龄、生长发育程度和父母体重水平等。这些变量作为第一批变量进入方程，解释了青少年体重水平9%的方差。研究数据还显示，"鼓励或强迫子女饮食"和"饮食和身体活动的监管"两种父母教养子女的行为分别解释了青少年体重水平的4.1%和1.1%的方差。而整个模型可以解释青少年 Z – BMI 共计14.2%的方差。

表 4.5　以父母教养子女的行为等变量预测青少年 Z－BMI 的
分层多元回归模型

| 预测变量 | B | β | 95% CI for B | Sig. | $R^2$（单独） |
|---|---|---|---|---|---|
| 第一步 | | | | | 0.089 |
| 青少年性别 | −0.425 | −0.113 | −0.677 － −0.173 | 0.001 | |
| 青少年年龄 | −0.293 | −0.135 | −0.453 － −0.134 | 0.000 | |
| 青少年生长发育程度 | 0.444 | 0.223 | 0.298 － 0.590 | 0.000 | |
| 父母体重水平 | 0.487 | 0.142 | 0.261 － 0.712 | 0.000 | |
| 第二步 | | | | | 0.042 |
| 鼓励或强迫子女饮食 | −0.231 | −0.274 | −0.297 － −0.165 | 0.000 | |
| 第三步 | | | | | 0.011 |
| 饮食和身体活动的监管 | 0.133 | 0.123 | 0.048 － 0.217 | 0.002 | |

Model $R^2$ : 0.143 ; Final multiple R = 0.378 , P < 0.01

备注：表格中仅列入了进入模型，具有统计学意义的变量

　　表 4.6 汇总了预测青少年饮食习惯的分层多元回归模型。第一步，性别和年龄解释了青少年饮食习惯 4% 的方差。而父母的"饮食和身体活动的监管"和"限制不健康饮食和静坐少动行为"则分别解释了 3.9% 和 0.9% 的方差变异。该模型共计解释了青少年饮食习惯 9% 的方差。

　　预测青少年身体活动的分层多元回归模型中，有性别、父亲受教育程度和家庭收入等变量被发现与青少年的身体活动水平有关，共计解释了 13% 的方差变异（表 4.7）。回归分析的结果还显示，父母的"饮食和身体活动的监管"行为解释了青少年身体活动水平方差变异的 1.3%。因此，该模型共计解释了青少年方差变异的 14.0%。

**表 4.6　以父母教养子女的行为等变量预测青少年饮食行为的分层多元回归模型**

| 预测变量 | B | β | 95% CI for B | Sig. | $R^2$（单独） |
|---|---|---|---|---|---|
| 第一步 | | | | | 0.046 |
| 青少年性别 | 1.470 | 0.371 | 0.742 – 2.198 | 0.000 | |
| 第二步 | | | | | 0.039 |
| 饮食和身体活动的监管 | 0.181 | 0.147 | 0.083 – 0.279 | 0.000 | |
| 第三步 | | | | | 0.009 |
| 限制不健康饮食和静坐少动行为 | 0.225 | 0.117 | 0.076 – 0.374 | 0.003 | |

Model $R^2$: 0.090; Final multiple R = 0.300, P < 0.01

备注：表格中仅列入了进入模型，具有统计学意义的变量

**表 4.7　以父母教养子女的行为等变量预测青少年身体活动水平的分层多元回归模型**

| 预测变量 | B | β | 95% CI for B | Sig. | $R^2$（单独） |
|---|---|---|---|---|---|
| 第一步 | | | | | 0.127 |
| 青少年性别 | −1.506 | −0.301 | −1.845 – −1.167 | 0.000 | |
| 父亲受教育程度 | 0.394 | 0.140 | 0.119 – 0.669 | 0.005 | |
| 家庭收入 | 0.375 | 0.086 | 0.077 – 0.699 | 0.014 | |
| 第二步 | | | | | 0.013 |
| 饮食和身体活动的监管 | 0.069 | 0.020 | 0.029 – 0.109 | 0.001 | |

Model $R^2$: 0.140; Final multiple R = 0.374, P < 0.01

备注：表格中仅列入了进入模型，具有统计学意义的变量

# 第四节　讨论与结论

本研究是国内为数不多的调查父母教养子女的行为与青少

年肥胖关系的研究之一。本次研究的数据发现，有几类父母教养子女的行为与青少年的 BMI、饮食习惯和身体活动水平有关，不过这些行为能够解释青少年的 BMI、饮食习惯和身体活动水平方差变异的百分比比较低。

"鼓励或强迫子女饮食"的行为是父母在抚养子女当中惯用的方法之一。先前的研究发现，这样的父母教养子女的行为对青少年的食物摄入和体重水平具有长期的影响（Clark, et al., 2007）。比如，有研究发现"鼓励或强迫子女饮食"的行为与青少年多吃蔬菜水果有关（Bourcier, et al., 2003）。一项横断面调查则发现父母"鼓励或强迫子女饮食"的行为可能对青少年的体重水平具有负面影响（Spruijt-Metz, et al., 2002）。另一项纵向跟踪研究则发现，父母会根据他们子女的体重水平来选择他们为子女提供食物的策略。该研究发现，对于瘦的子女，父母更倾向于采用"鼓励或强迫子女饮食"的行为，也更少控制子女的饮食（Lee, et al., 2001）。本次研究的结果也证实了该研究结果。本次研究的数据显示，父母"鼓励或强迫子女饮食"的行为与青少年的 BMI（$r = -0.22, p < 0.01$）和 Z – BMI（$r = -0.23, p < 0.01$）均呈负相关。此外，回归分析的结果还发现，父母"鼓励或强迫子女饮食"的行为可以解释青少年体重水平 4.2% 的方差。而另一项研究则发现父母"鼓励或强迫子女饮食"的行为以及父母对青少年体重问题的关注可以解释青少年总脂肪量 15% 的方差（Spruijt-Metz, et al., 2002）。由于在 Spruijt-Mets 等人的研究中，两项父母行为在同一批进入模型，因此无法比较该研究与本研究的数据。但是，两项研究的结果

都显示，父母"鼓励或强迫子女饮食"的行为与青少年体重水平有关。

有研究发现"禁止青少年食用某种食物"和"把食物当作青少年的奖励"与青少年的食物摄入有关（Rhee，2008）。比如，有研究报道了"禁止青少年食用某种食物"的行为存在一些负面效应。相反，青少年的体重水平也会影响父母是否采用这类教养行为（Fisher & Birch，1999a）。本次研究发现，父母的"禁止青少年食用某种食物"的行为与青少年的饮食行为有关。回归分析也发现，父母"限制不健康饮食和静坐少动行为"是影响青少年饮食习惯的变量之一。此外，数据还显示，父母对青少年饮食和身体活动的监管也与青少年饮食习惯有关，这也与前人的研究结果一致（Lindsay，et al.，2006；Rhee，2008）。不过，值得注意的是，这些行为能够解释青少年饮食习惯方差的比例不高。

充足的身体活动被认为是控制体重最重要的手段之一（Jakicic & Otto，2005）。目前的研究发现，父母教养子女的行为会影响青少年身体活动水平。比如，与父母身体活动不积极的青少年相比，父母身体活动积极的青少年积极参与身体活动的概率更高（Moore，et al.，1991）。还有的研究发现，得到父母更多支持的青少年要比较少获得父母支持的青少年更积极地投身身体活动（O'Loughlin，et al.，1999）。但是这些研究的结果也不尽相同。比如，有研究发现，女生们的身体活动与父母报告的对子女参与身体活动的支持程度相关，但是却与女生们感受到的父母支持程度不相关（Adkins，et al.，2004）。另一项研究则发现，对子女参与身体活动的支持程度与青少年自我主观报告的身体活动水平相关，但与加速器测量的客观青少年身体活动水平不相关（Prochaska, et al., 2002）。在本次研究中，我们发现，"限制不健康饮食和静坐少动行为"和"饮食和身体活动的监管"两种父母教养子女的行为与青少年身体活动水平显著相关。但是，分层多元回归模型的结果也显示，这些行为仅能解释青少年身体活动水平方差变异的比例比较低。本次研究的数据提示，父母教养子女的行为可能与青少年身体活动水平存在具有统计学意义的微弱相关。

此外，本研究并没有发现父亲和母亲在父母教养子女的方式上存在大的差异，仅在某几项教养方式上存在具有统计学意义的微弱差异。很长时间，中国家庭受到儒家思想影响，妇女在家庭中地位卑微（S. W. K. Yu & Chau, 1997）。但是，自从1979 年施行独生子女政策后，中国家庭中的父权制受到了挑战。近年来的研究也显示，在施行独生子女政策后我国妇女地位也得到了明显改善（Deutsch, 2006）。因此，在过去30 多年，中国家庭男女逐渐平等可能可以部分解释为什么在本研究中父母在子女教养行为上仅有微弱差异。

另一方面，20 世纪70 年代施行独生子女政策后，许多中国家庭的父母教养子女的行为和方式也发生了改变（Jing, 1994）。许多中国孩子在家里被父母当作了小皇帝、小女王，这与传统的中国父母教养子女的方式差异明显。比如，父母为了表达他们对子女的爱，常常在吃饭时给子女夹菜。有研究发现，56%的父母常常提醒他们的子女多吃点他们认为健康的食品，甚至有7.7%的父母常常强迫子女吃这些食品（W. J. Ma, et al., 2001）。本次研究的结果也显示，"鼓励或强迫子女饮食"是中国父母常采用的行为，这与中国传统家庭中，父亲专制、严厉的形象不同。鉴于"鼓励或强迫子女饮食"可能影响青少年自身调节能量摄入的能力，这种行为可能导致青少年过量摄取能量，并最终导致肥胖。本研究也提示，在针对青少年肥胖问题的干预中，不仅应考虑父母的行为，还应考虑到父母的理念。

需要说明的是，本次研究还存在一些不足。首先，本次研究采用的是横断面调查研究，因此不能确定变量之间的因果关系。其他的不足还包括自我报告式的数据调查方式、抽样样本不具有全国代表性等。本次研究的优势则包括较大的样本量和经过完善信度、效度测试的调查问卷。

综上所述，本次研究的结果显示，青少年的体重水平、饮食习惯和身体活动与一些父母的教养行为存在具有统计学意义的微弱相关。这些父母教养子女的行为包括：鼓励或强迫子女饮食、饮食和身体活动的监管、限制不健康饮食和静坐少动行为等等。但是，研究结果也显示父亲和母亲在教养行为上不存在较大差异。

# 第五章 中国父母对其子女体重的认知与教养子女行为的关系研究

## 第一节 前　言

儿童肥胖问题在当今世界越来越凸显。不论是发达国家还是发展中国家儿童肥胖率与日俱增。中国的营养问题也已经从儿童青少年的营养不良转变为营养过剩（Y. Wang, et al., 2002）。对 1989 - 1997 年中国城市地区的调查发现，儿童 2 - 6 岁肥胖率从先前的 1.5% 增加到 12.6%，超重的成年人从14.6% 增长到 28.6%。（Luo & Hu, 2002）

专家们建议父母及其子女通过改变饮食习惯并进行体育锻炼的措施来预防儿童肥胖（Barlow & the Expert Committee, 2007）。父母在儿童形成饮食习惯和体育锻炼倾向性方面有重要的影响（Rhee, 2008）。因此，父母通过改变其教养子女的方式方法来帮助孩子减肥的意愿是极其关键的。健康信念模式表明决定个体健康相关行为的一个重要因素是其认识到特定的健康问题对自身健康构成威胁的程度（Elder, et al., 1999；Janz &

Becker, 1984；Rhee, 2008）。因此，父母在认识到孩子的体重问题之前或许是不太愿意改变其行为的。当前的研究也证实了父母对儿童体重的认识与其帮助儿童减肥的意愿之间的关系（Rhee, et al., 2005）。

然而，欧洲和美国的研究表明，有相当高比例的父母不能准确认识子女的体重（Eckstein, et al., 2006；Etelson, et al., 2003；Ward, 2008）。比如，在美国一项代表性的研究表明，近乎80%的母亲不能意识到其子女已经超重（Baughcum, et al., 2000）。在德国开展的一项调查发现，只有40.3%的母亲能准确地认识其子女的体重（Warschburger & Kroller, 2009）。在中国，针对父母对孩子体重的了解程度也展开了一些调查（Shi, et al., 2007；Xie, et al., 2006）。约22%父母认为其正常体重的子女体重偏轻，23%的父母认为其超重的孩子是正常体重。（Shi, et al., 2007）

近来的研究中，学者们广泛地讨论了父母对其子女体重认识程度的影响因素。儿童及其父母的因素，包括儿童的体重、年龄、性别和父母的体重、受教育程度和家庭收入被认为与父母对子女体重的认识程度有关联（Baughcum, et al., 2000；Campbell, et al., 2006；Huang, et al., 2007；Warschburger & Kroller, 2009）。一些研究明确提出了父母教养子女的行为与儿童肥胖存在相关（Birch & Fisher, 1998；Faith, Scanlon, et al., 2004；Rhee, 2008），但是现在的研究中父母对其子女体重的认识程度与促进健康饮食和体育锻炼等的教养子女行为之间的直接关系却少有涉及（Hodges, 2003）。此外，尽管很多研究中都涉及中国青少年及父母的体重认知（Shi, et al., 2007; Xie, et al., 2006; Xie, et al., 2003），但这些研究往往侧重于青少年自我体重的认识和满意度。目前还未开展父母对其子女体重认识的相关研究。因此，本研究的目的是调查中国父母对其子女的体重认知，并研究父母教养子女的行为与对子女体重水平认识的关系。

## 第二节　研究方法

### 研究对象与方案

本文调查对象的选取为中国南方的两个城市的青少年及其父母，因为与农村地区相比，城市地区存在肥胖问题更严重（Luo & Hu, 2002）。由于经济和社会发展与人们的高热量食物摄入、静坐少动行为、肥胖超重问题有关（Y. Wang, et al., 2002），因此本研究决定在我国南方的发达地区和欠发达地区分别抽取研究对象。研究采用随机分层抽样法，抽取汕头市作为南方发达地区代表，赣州市作为南方欠发达地区代表。汕头是我国 20 世纪 80 年代最早建立的经济特区之一。根据 2010 年汕头市政府统计公报的数据，汕头市 2010 年人均 GDP 为 20279 元（Shantou municipal bureau of statistics, 2010）。赣州作为我国的革命老区，是一个欠发达的内陆城市。根据 2010 年赣州市政府统计公报的数据，赣州市人 2010 年人均 GDP 为 9391 元。

研究随机选取这两个城市初中一年级和二年级的青少年及其父母作为调查对象。以赣州为例，赣州有两个行政区。在本研究中，在每个区抽取一所重点中学和一所普通中学，每所中学抽取 4 到 6 个班级（每个年级 2－3 个班）。同样的抽样策略也应用于汕头市。青少年如果曾接受过可能影响其体重的治疗，或者存在身体残疾或慢性病，不能作为本研究的研究对象。

在 2009 年 4 月到 5 月，有 2162 组青少年及其父母参与了本次调查（其中赣州 1179 组，汕头 1106 组），其中 19 位青少年由于存在身体残疾或需要接受药物治疗会影响其体重，所以不将其纳入研究分析。在调查过程中，274 位家长未交回调查问卷，最终有 2143 位青少年以及 1869 位家长的调查数据被纳入数据分析。

在调查中，青少年们需要完成身高与体重的测量，然后在教室填写一份问卷，如有需要调查人员将提供帮助。然后青少年要将新的问卷带回家让其父母填写（父亲或母亲都可以填写问卷）。随后问卷将统一由调查人员收集，调查人员会向被调查者送上小礼物以示感谢。

另有 127 组青少年及其父母（赣州 62 组，汕头 65 组）在开展调查前四周对问卷进行可靠性检验，相隔两周重复完成这份问卷。问卷的再测信度和内在一致性通过同类相关系数和克隆巴赫系数分别进行验证。

在调查之前需要获得调查对象的署名同意。父母被引导提供关于其子女健康状况的信息，并鼓励青少年及父母按真实想法作答。在问卷调查中，答案不分对错，而且调查人员将对问卷严格保密。研究获得了香港中文大学研究伦理委员会的正式许可。

### 主要调查内容

#### 青少年体重状况

对青少年体重的测量精确到 0.1 千克（脱鞋、着最少的衣服），身高测量精确到 0.5 厘米。并计算出体重指数（BMI），计算公式为 $BMI = 体重（kg）/身高（m）^2$，其标准定为偏瘦（低于同性别同年龄段儿童群体平均值两个标准差）、正常或超重（高于同性别同年龄段儿童群体平均值一个标准差），该标准是世界健康组织（WHO）根据世界青少年（学生时期青少年）成长标准制定的（Butte, et al., 2007; De Onis, et al., 2007）。

#### 父母体重状况

父母的 BMI 指数是通过其问卷中的身高、体重计算得出（因为测量父母的身高体重可行性较低）。问卷中填写的身高体重的信度将得到验证。（Bolton-Smith et al. 2000; Wada et al. 2005）调查对象的问卷 BMI 值与测量值的皮尔森相关系数分别为男性 0.943 和女性 0.950（Wada et al. 2005）。成人的 BMI 值标准为不超重（$BMI < 24kg/m^2$），超重（$24kg/m^2 \leqslant BMI < 28kg/m^2$），肥胖（$BMI \geqslant 28kg/m^2$）（Zhou & Cooperative Meta-Analysis Group of the Working Group on Obesity in China, 2002），作为判断中国成年人超重或肥胖的 BMI 值标准。

#### 父母对其子女的体重的认知情况

父母需要回答其子女的体重情况，有五个选项分别是"体重太轻"、"偏轻"、"正常"、"偏重"、"非常超重"来评价他们对子女体重的观察。然后分级定为"体重不足"（"体重太轻"、

"偏轻")、"体重正常"("正常")、"超重"("偏重"、"非常超重")三个等级来进一步分析。此项的再测信度为0.88。

**青少年对自身体重的认知情况**

由学者 Collins 提出的直观图是用来检验青少年对自身体重的认识情况(Collins, 1991)。它由 7 幅图构成,人的体型从极瘦到极胖。青少年被问及"哪一幅图最能代表现在你的体型?"并从 7 幅图中进行选择。此项的再测信度为 0.71 (Collins, 1991)。从信度检验的结果看再测信度为 0.92。然后再将分级定为"体重不足"("体重太轻"、"偏轻")、"体重正常"("正常")、"超重"("偏重"、"非常超重")三个等级来分析(Warschburger & Kroller, 2009)。选择最左边的两个图定义为"体重不足",选择随后的三个图被定义为"体重正常",选择最后两个图被定义为"体重超重"。父母对其子女以及青少年自身体重的认知与真实体重进行比较,将其进行"对"或"错"的区分。

**父母对子女的教养行为**

采用 17 项的李克特五点量表,这一问卷是在原有研究基础上进行修改和翻译得出的(Arredondo, et al., 2006; O'Connor, et al., 2010),用于评价父母对子女的教养行为。这一量表包括以下子项目"饮食及体育活动的监督","用食物或静态行为作为奖励","饮食的控制压力","限制不健康的食物和静态行为"和"青少年的饮食习惯和身体活动的巩固"。李克特五点量表提供可能的选项分别是:从不、极少、有时、经常、总是或者非常不同意、不同意、不确定、同意、非常同意。父母的教养行为各个子项数据相加得出总分。有遗漏的数据用其他教养行为的平均值代替。在父母教养子女的行为子项中最高的遗漏数据百分比为0.9%。在调查中获得的数据需要验证其效度。本研究选用 LISREL 8.51 版统计软件进行实证的因子分析，关于问卷的信度和效度，请查阅表 3.3 和表 3.6。

**其他数据**

从问卷中获得青少年的性别和年龄，由其父母提供背景材料比如受教育程度、父母年龄以及家庭收入。

**数据分析**

采用 Kappa 统计检验父母对其子女体重的认知与实际体重的一致性。采用多元回归分析预测影响父母认知的影响因素。采用单因素方差分析比较对子女体重能正确认知和不能正确认知的父母其教养行为得出的不同数值。比较变量（如青少年体重状况、性别、年龄）对父母教养子女的行为的影响。

# 第三节 结 果

本次研究共收集到 2143 名青少年和 1869 名家长的调查数据。关于受试对象的基本信息如表 5.1 所示。

表 5.1 受试对象基本情况（N = 2143）

| 青少年性别, % | |
| --- | --- |
| 男生 | 51.4 |
| 女生 | 48.6 |

| | |
|---|---|
| 青少年年龄，平均值 ± 标准差，岁 | 12.5 ± 0.9 |
| 青少年体重水平，% | |
| 　体重偏低 | 2.4 |
| 　正常 | 80.9 |
| 　超重 | 16.7 |
| 青少年 BMI，平均值 ± 标准差 | 18.6 ± 2.8 |
| 青少年饮食习惯，平均值 ± 标准差 | 39.3 ± 5.3 |
| 青少年身体活动水平，平均值 ± 标准差 | 5.1 ± 2.8 |
| 父母性别，% | |
| 　男性 | 40.4 |
| 　女性 | 59.6 |
| 父母 BMI，平均值 ± 标准差 | 22.2 ± 3.0 |
| 父母教养子女的行为，平均值 ± 标准差 | |
| 　饮食和身体活动的监控 | 19.8 ± 4.3 |
| 　把食物或静坐少动行为当作奖励 | 5.4 ± 1.8 |
| 　鼓励或强迫子女饮食 | 9.8 ± 2.1 |
| 　限制不健康饮食和静坐少动行为 | 15.4 ± 2.7 |
| 　对子女健康饮食和身体活动的鼓励 | 7.0 ± 2.1 |
| 地区，% | |
| 　赣州 | 45.7 |
| 　汕头 | 54.3 |

　　研究数据表明 2/5 的父母不能正确认知其子女的体重状况，并且接近 3/5 的青少年不能正确地认知自己的体重状况。如表 5.2 所示，青少年实际 BMI 值与父母对其体重的认知一致

性很低（Kappa = 0.221）。近 40% 的父母认为其超重的子女体重为正常或偏轻。有 42.2% 的父母认为其正常体重的子女偏瘦。同时，青少年实际 BMI 值与自己体重的认知一致性也很低（Kappa = 0.167）。约 30% 的超重青少年认为自己是正常体重或体重偏轻。此外，55.0% 正常体重的青少年认为自己偏瘦。

**表 5.2　青少年体重水平与其父母对子女体重水平认知的一致性**

| | 青少年的 BMI 水平（N，%） | | | kappa |
| --- | --- | --- | --- | --- |
| | 偏瘦 | 正常 | 超重 | |
| 父母的认知 | | | | 0.221 |
| 偏瘦 | 44（91.7） | 626（42.2） | 6（1.9） | |
| 正常 | 2（4.2） | 802（54.1） | 120（38.5） | |
| 超重 | 2（4.2） | 55（3.7） | 186（59.6） | |
| 青少年的自我认知 | | | | 0.167 |
| 偏瘦 | 44（84.6） | 949（55.0） | 21（5.9） | |
| 正常 | 8（15.4） | 635（36.8） | 90（25.3） | |
| 超重 | 0（0） | 141（8.2） | 245（68.8） | |

备注：由于数据不完整，有 10 名青少年和 26 名父母的数据未进入青少年体重水平与其父母对子女体重水平认知的一致性分析。

　　研究数据表明一些因素将影响父母对子女的体重认知（见表 5.3）。相比而言，中国父母判断男孩的体重比女孩更为不准确［比值（OR）= 1.61，95% 置信区间（CI）为 1.29 – 2.01］，其中母亲对子女体重判断更为准确（OR = 0.80，CI：0.64 – 1.00）。回归分析的结果页得出父母对其体重的认知与青少年自身的体重认知存在关联。能正确判断自身体重的青少年其父母也能更准确地判断体重情况（OR = 0.30，CI：0.24 – 0.38）。其他青少年及父母的情况不存在显著的联系。

表 5.3　影响父母误判子女体重水平相关因素的 logistic 回归分析

| | | 调整后 OR（95% CI） |
| --- | --- | --- |
| 青少年的性别 | 女孩 | 参考对象 |
| | 男孩 | 1.61（1.29 – 2.01）** |
| 青少年对自身体重的认知 | 不正确 | 参考对象 |
| | 正确 | 0.30（0.24 – 0.38）** |
| 父母的性别 | 父亲 | 参考对象 |
| | 母亲 | 0.80（0.64 – 1.00）* |
| 家庭子女的人数 | 1 | 参考对象 |
| | ≥2 | 0.99（0.72 – 1.35） |
| 父母的体重水平 | 正常 | 参考对象 |
| | 超重 | 0.98（0.75 – 1.28） |
| | 肥胖 | 0.66（0.37 – 1.20） |
| 父母教育水平 | 初中或以下 | 参考对象 |
| | 高中 | 0.94（0.70 – 1.27） |
| | 大学或以上 | 0.70（0.53 – 1.10） |
| 家庭收入 | 低 | 参考对象 |
| | 中 | 0.94（0.73 – 1.19） |
| | 高 | 0.88（0.48 – 1.60） |
| 地域 | 赣州 | 参考对象 |
| | 汕头 | 1.18（0.86 – 1.62） |

备注：logistic 回归分析控制了青少年年龄和体重的影响；*：$P < .05$；**：$P < .01$

**表 5.4  对子女体重水平有正确和错误认知的父母教养子女行为的差异**

| | 父母教养子女的行为的平均分 (95% CI) | | ANCOVA Test | | |
|---|---|---|---|---|---|
| | 正确 | 错误 | F | p | Cohen's d |
| 饮食和身体活动的监管 | 20.38 (20.05 – 20.71) | 19.52 (19.15 – 19.89) | 11.93 | 0.001 | 0.20 |
| 把食物或静坐少动行为当作奖励 | 5.62 (5.48 – 5.76) | 5.52 (5.36 – 5.67) | 0.58 | 0.447 | 0.06 |
| 鼓励或强迫子女饮食 | 9.69 (9.53 – 9.86) | 10.12 (10.01 – 10.38) | 20.26 | 0.000 | 0.21 |
| 限制不健康饮食和静坐少动行为 | 15.56 (15.34 – 15.78) | 15.35 (15.10 – 15.59) | 1.62 | 0.204 | 0.08 |
| 对子女健康饮食和身体活动的鼓励 | 7.20 (7.04 – 7.36) | 6.95 (6.77 – 7.13) | 4.05 | 0.044 | 0.12 |

备注：数据分析控制了青少年体重、性别以及年龄的影响。

　　父母教养子女的行为与子女的肥胖状况存在联系，研究通过父母能正确判断其子女体重与不能做出正确判断采用协因素方差分析进行比较（表5.4）。研究数据表明能正确认知子女体重的父母与不能正确认知的父母存在显著性差异，尽管效应值很小。正确认知子女体重的父母在监督子女的饮食和身体活动方面分值更高（$P < 0.01$），对其子女健康饮食和身体活动也给予更多的鼓励（$P < 0.05$）。不能正确判断其子女体重的父母更易于鼓励或强迫子女饮食（$P < 0.01$）。然而在"把食物或静坐少动行为当作奖励"和"限制不健康饮食和静坐少动行为"这两项父母教养子女的行为上，正确判断与不能正确判断子女体重水平的父母之间并不存在具有统计学意义的差别。

# 第四节 讨 论

本研究显示 16.7% 的青少年超重，超过 1/4 的父母超重或肥胖。在中国，青少年的肥胖问题越来越凸显，成为公共健康的主要问题之一（Ji & Working Group on Obesity in China, 2005），尽管其普遍程度还不及发达国家。研究表明，父母对子女体重认知与青少年实际体重之间的一致性较低。本次研究中家长不能正确判断其子女体重相比 2002 年数据的比例更大（Shi, et al., 2007）（见表 5.2）。出现这一结果的原因可能是两次研究时间的不同或两次研究采用的不同研究方法（抽样涉及和测量设备）。本次研究显示只有 56% 的家长能够正确判断其子女的体重状况，这与其他研究得出的结果相似。在美国的一项研究显示，只有 60% 的母亲正确判断了其子女体重（Boutelle, Fulkerson, Neumark-Sztainer, & Story, 2004）。中国父母也不能更准确地判断其子女的体重，尽管研究表明其准确度受种族的影响（Boutelle, Fulkerson, Neumark-Sztainer, & Story, 2004）。此外，本研究采用了国际卫生组织（WHO）制订的生长参考数据作为青少年肥胖判断的标准。在该标准中，19 岁男生 BMI 平均值加一个标准差的临界值是 25.4kg/m$^2$，而 19 岁女生相应的临界值为 25kg/m$^2$（De Onis et al. 2007）。值得注意的是这一标准是与成年人超重标准相联系的，而中国成年人通常采用的超重标准为 24kg/m$^2$（Zhou & Cooperative Meta-Analysis Group of the Working Group on Obesity in China, 2002）。因此，如果采用更为严格的青少年超重标准，则父母对子女体重的错误判断比例会更大。

父母对子女体重的判断与父母和子女的特性也存在联系（Huang，et al.，2007）。研究结果表明父母对子女体重的判断和青少年自身体重判断都与性别有关。比起男孩，超重的女孩更能引起其母亲的关注（Campbell，et al.，2006；Maynard，Galuska，Blanck，& Serdula，2003）。中国父母也较易错误判断男孩的体重。母亲更能正确辨别子女的体重，这一性别差异的原因可能源于社会价值观念（Campbell，et al.，2006）。比如，较为瘦小的身材的女孩更为社会所认可，而超重的男孩则常常被认为更强壮、健康而不是肥胖。因此，中国父母对女孩体重的关注比男孩更为密切，而在美国和澳大利亚情况同样如此（Campbell，et al.，2006；Maynard，et al.，2003）。

到目前为止，父母不能正确判断其子女体重的现象还未得出原因。原因可能是父母对子女正确的体重认知能力较低，或不能明确辨别"超重"和"肥胖"的概念，或是情绪原因父母不愿承认子女超重或肥胖（Maynard，et al.，2003）。质化研究表明低收入的美国家庭母亲宁愿认为其超重的子女强壮而不愿认为其超重或肥胖（Jain，et al.，2001）。最近的研究表明社会经济状况与母亲对自己子女体重的认知无关，而与非自己子女的超重情况认知有关（Warschburger & Kroller，2009）。因此，母亲对自己子女的认知更多受情绪因素的影响而不是对肥胖程度、体型的认知等与教育水平相关因素的影响。研究还显示父母对子女的体重认知与性别相关，而与父母的教育水平和家庭收入不存在关联。与本研究结果相似的是，父母对子女体重的认知更多由于情感因素，并与父母和青少年的性别有关，而不是教育水平、家庭收入、家庭中的孩子数量等因素有关。然而，本研究尚未能证实这一假设，需要通过以后的研究进一步探析其原因。

健康信念模型认为最初通过行为改变进行体重控制的动机水平来自于对肥胖的威胁程度（Daddario，2007）。因此，纠正青少年及其父母对青少年体重水平的认知错误可能是体重控制最初阶段很重要的一步。先前的研究表明，青少年及其父母低估其体重状况与不良饮食习惯和健康饮食习惯以及锻炼习惯存在障碍有关（Skinner, Weinberger, Mulvaney, Schlundt, & Rothman，2008）。而且，青少年对自身超重问题的反馈将影响父母改变其教养子女行为的意愿（Warschburger & Kroller，2009）。通过研究学校的重量筛选干预心理因素给予父母反馈，结果表明这一反馈不会影响正常体重子女的父母改变其教养方式。然而，超重女孩的父母会对其施加更严格的饮食控制（Grimmett, Croker, Carnell, & Wardle，2008）。另一个横截面研究表明正确地区分超重的青少年不会导致有益的行为，而可能会引起不健康的行为，比如增加饮食（Neumark-Sztainer, Wall, Story, & van den Berg，2008）。近来研究表明一些教养子女的行为，比如"饮食和身体活动的监管"、"鼓励或强迫子女饮食"、"对子女健康饮食和身体活动的鼓励"都与父母对其子女的体重认知有关。这些教养行为也已被证实导致儿童肥胖（Birch & Fisher，1998；Rhee，2008）。比如，一些研究表明父母"鼓励或强迫子女饮食"的方式与青少年卡路里摄入有关（Drucker, Hammer, Agras, & Bryson, 1999），还与脂肪摄入有关（Spruijt-Metz, Lindquist, Birch, Fisher, & Goran, 2002）。最近的研究表明能正确认知其子女体重状况的父母一般不会经常使用"鼓励或强迫子女饮食"的方法，尽管此项的效应值不高，但这一现象不能被忽视（Pedersen, 2003）。结果表明正确的体重认知与积极的教养行为有关，而这也有助于青少年预防肥胖。

本研究结果还表明青少年对自身体重的认知与其父母对子女体重认知有关。另一项研究对 718 名青少年及其父母进行调查，发现父母对子女的体重认知会影响青少年对自身的体重认知（Huang, Donohue, Becerra, & Xu, 2009）。这些研究结果表明父母对其子女体重认知与教养子女行为有关，也与青少年对自身体重认知有关，而这些都将对青少年肥胖问题产生影响。

本研究也存在一些不足之处。其一，本研究采用 BMI 值进行体重分类而非身体脂肪含量。尽管采用不同年龄段的 BMI 值对超重和肥胖儿童的检测更为有效（Ji & Working Group on Obesity in China, 2005; Mei, et al., 2002）。本研究在体重分类时可能存在误差，因为 BMI 值并不能直接代替体脂含量。其二，采用 Collins 不同体型的图形让青少年判断自身的体重状况，并不是基于某个 BMI 范围内男生或女生的实际图片描绘的。不过，Collins 的图形与学者 Warschburger 和 Kroller 基于特定的学龄前儿童 BMI 值说创设的图形很相似（Warschburger & Kroller, 2009）。这一分类方法也在应用于本次研究，尽管其中也存在不足之处。研究结果也不适用于所有的中国人，因为样本抽取中国南方的城市地区。其他不足在于对结果解释的不足，包括自我报告的真实性和横截面研究的设计。

　　尽管存在一些不足，但本研究还是证实了对青少年体重水平的错误认知是中国父母的普遍现象。父母对其子女体重的认知的正确性与性别和青少年对自身体重认知情况有关。父母对子女的体重认知和父母教养子女的行为相关的结果表明，青少年体重的准确分类可以预防青少年肥胖问题。

# 第六章　父母教养子女的方式是父母教养子女的行为与青少年体重水平的调节变量

## 第一节　前　言

青少年肥胖问题已经成为发达国家日益严重的公共卫生问题（Lehingue，1999；Ogden，et al.，2002）。在过去的 10 年，中国青少年的肥胖问题也发展迅速（Ji & Working Group on Obesity in China，2005）。父母在青少年肥胖的发展和预防中发挥着重要作用。有研究发现，青少年肥胖可能与父母的教养行为有关（Clark，et al.，2007）。比如，父母喂养儿童，或为青少年提供食物的行为可能直接影响青少年的饮食习惯和对食物的偏爱，也可能影响青少年调节能量摄入的能力，最终影响他们的体重水平（Nguyen，et al.，1996）。此外，近期的研究还发现，青少年的体重问题可能与他们父母的教养子女的方式有关（Rhee，et al.，2006）。

父母教养子女的方式是指父母在教育和抚养孩子的行为表

达的态度和所创造的情感环境（Darling & Steinberg, 1993）。目前，应用最为广泛的父母教养子女的方式理论最早建立于 20 世纪 70 年代。根据该理论，父母教养子女的方式的相关研究通常以关爱（responsiveness）和控制（demandingness）两个维度为出发点，把父母分成 4 种教养方式：民主型（高关爱、高控制）、专制型（低关爱、高控制）、溺爱型（高关爱、低控制）与放任型（低关爱、低控制）（Baumrind, 1971）。由于父母的教养方式为青少年的成长和父母教养子女的行为的表达提供了环境和情感上的背景，因此，父母教养子女的方式可能对于青少年肥胖的预防非常重要。有几项研究调查了父母教养子女的方式与青少年肥胖的关系。如有研究发现，与民主型母亲的孩子相比，专制型、溺爱型和放任型母亲所抚养的孩子更容易发生肥胖问题（Rhee, et al., 2006）。另一项来自澳大利亚的纵向跟踪研究则报道，父亲教养子女的方式可能与儿童肥胖有关（Wake, et al., 2007）。此外，一项基于 163 名华裔青少年（8 - 10 岁）及其母亲的研究还发现，民主型教养方式与青少年的 BMI 呈正比（J. L. Chen & Kennedy, 2004）。但是，目前的研究还未厘清父母教养子女的方式影响青少年体重水平的机制。

另一方面，值得考虑的是父母教养子女的方式可能存在的文化差异。虽然 Baumrind（1971）所建立的父母教养子女的方式理论已经广泛应用于中国人群（X. Y. Chen, et al., 1997；Pong, et al., 2009；Porter, et al., 2005），有学者仍认为中国父母教养子女的方式可能更偏向于民主型和专制型（Xu, et al., 2005）。此外，针对父母教养子女的方式的测量没有标准的临界值，4 种父母教养子女的方式的分类依靠相对标准（比如：中位数）。这可能导致在不同的族群，用于父母教养子女的方式的分类的临界值千差万别。因此，采用父母教养子女的方式关爱和控制两个维度的连续变量，而不是 4 种父母教子女的方式的分类变量研究中国父母的教养方式可能更为合理。

Darling 和 Steinberg（1993）提出的假说认为，父母的教养方式是影响父母行为与青少年反应关系的调节变量。根据该父母教养子女的方式的理论模型，父母的教养子女方式可能可以加强父母教养子女的行为对青少年体重水平的影响。Van der Horst 等人（2007）的研究也证实了父母教养子女的方式可以调节父母教养子女的行为与青少年含糖饮料的摄入。但是，关于父母教养子女的方式调节父母教养子女的行为和青少年体重水平的研究鲜有报道。

因此，根据 Darling 和 Steinberg 建立的理论模型，本次研究的目的是确定父母教养子女的方式是否是影响父母教养子女的行为和青少年饮食习惯、身体活动水平和体重水平关系的调节变量。

# 第二节　研究方法

### 研究对象与方案

因为与农村地区相比，城市地区肥胖问题更严重（Luo & Hu, 2002），本文调查对象的选取为中国南方的两个城市的青少年及其父母。研究采用随机分层抽样法，抽取汕头市作为南方发达地区代表，赣州市作为南方欠发达地区代表。研究随机选取这两个城市初中一年级和二年级的青少年以及其父母作为调查对象。在本研究中，在两座城市各随机选取两个行政区，在每个区抽取一所重点中学和一所普通中学，每所中学抽取4到6个班级（每个年级2－3个班）。在2009年4月到5月，有2162组青少年及其父母参与了本次调查（其中赣州1179组、汕头1106组）。调查对象中超过99%为汉族。研究对象中19位青少年由于存在身体残疾或需要接受药物治疗会影响其体重所以不将其纳入研究分析。在调查过程中，274位家长未交回调查问卷，最终有2143位青少年以及1869位家长的调查数据最终被纳入数据分析。

在调查中，青少年们需要完成身高与体重的测量，然后在教室填写一份问卷，如有需要调查人员将提供帮助。然后青少年要将新的问卷带回家让其父母填写（父亲或母亲都可以填写问卷）。随后问卷将统一由调查人员收集，调查人员会向被调查者送上小礼物以示感谢。

另有127组青少年及其父母（赣州62组，汕头65组）在开展调查前四周对问卷进行可靠性检验，相隔两周重复完成这份问卷。问卷的再测信度和内在一致性通过同类相关系数和克隆巴赫系数分别进行验证。

在调查之前需要获得调查对象的署名同意。父母被引导提供关于其子女健康状况的信息并鼓励青少年及父母按真实想法作答。研究获得了香港中文大学研究伦理委员会的正式许可。

### 主要调查指标

#### 青少年的年龄、性别和体重水平

青少年的年龄、性别信息是通过青少年问卷中受试对象的报告获取。对青少年体重的测量精确到 0.1 千克（脱鞋、穿尽量少的衣服），身高测量精确到 0.5 厘米。计算出经过性别和年龄调整后的体重指数 Z 分（Z - BMI），Z - BMI 的计算根据世界健康组织（WHO）学龄青少年成长标准（Butte, et al., 2007; De Onis, et al., 2007）。

#### 青少年的饮食习惯

采用 12 项的李克特五点量表测量青少年的饮食习惯。在调查中，青少年通过五个回答选项（"从不"、"很少"、"有时"、"经常"和"总是"）来回答关于他们饮食行为习惯的问题。问题例子："我每天吃至少三份水果"、"假如饭菜味道好，我会多吃一点"。有研究显示，该问卷具有良好的可靠性和有效性（Sheu, 2003）。本研究的可靠性测试显示，该问卷题目的两周重复性信度为 0.70 - 0.79，问卷的内部一致性为 0.71。

#### 青少年的身体活动水平

受试青少年被邀请填写儿童青少年身体活动水平问卷（PARCY）以评价他们过去一年的每周平均活动水平。PARCY 是在 Jackson Activity Coding 问卷（Baumgartner & Jackson, 1996; George, et al., 1997）和 Godin-Shephard Activity Questionnaire 问卷（Aaron, et al., 1993; Godin & Shephard, 1985）的基础上改编的单问题量表。PARCY 问卷的效标效度和同证效度也已经被其他一些研究所证实（Hui, 2001; Hui, et al., 2001; Kong, et al.,

2010）。PARCY 问卷是一个 11 分（0 – 10 级）的量表，0 级为完全没有任何身体活动，而 10 级为每天都有大量剧烈身体活动。本次研究的可靠性测试显示，该量表的两周重测信度为 0.83。

### 青少年发育程度

虽然有许多研究已经发现青少年的肥胖程度与其发育时间密切相关（Kaplowitz, et al., 2001；Tremblay & Frigon, 2005），但是目前对于青少年肥胖的研究并没有很好地控制青少年发育程度对研究结果的影响（Tsiros, et al., 2008）。在本次研究中，采用了一个自评问卷，请青少年报告他们的阴毛、性器官、乳房（仅针对女生）发育情况，以确定青少年的发育程度。有研究发现该问卷测量青少年发育状况具有良好的可靠性（Chan, et al., 2008）。本研究的前期研究发现，该问卷两个题目的两周重测信度分别为 0.80 和 0.82，内部一致性为 0.71。

### 青少年报告的父母教养子女的方式

受试青少年被要求通过回答父母 API 问卷（Authoritative Parenting Index）中的问题报告他们父亲和母亲的教养方式。

父母 API 问卷的结构与父母教养子女的方式的理论模型一致，并具有较好的信度（Jackson, et al., 1998）。API 问卷共有 16 个题目，其中有 9 个关于父母关爱的题目，另 7 个关于父母控制的题目。API 问卷英文版由两位通晓中英双语的研究者翻译后，再由另两位研究者回译，以保证问卷翻译质量。前期研究证明该问卷题目的两周重测信度为 0.70 到 0.85。而问卷的两个亚量表在父亲和母亲中的内部一致性为 0.70 到 0.75。同时，以本次调查的数据为基础，采用 LISREL 8.51 软件和验证性因子分析的方法，计算了问卷的结构效度。研究数据显示，问卷每个题目的载荷处于可接受水平，针对父亲受试对象的题目载荷范围为 0.55 到 0.76，在母亲受试者则为 0.59 到 0.74。拟合指数 RMSEA，CFI 和 NNFI 的计算结果则显示，问卷符合理论模型（基于父亲们的数据 RMSEA = 0.056，NNFI = 0.92，CFI = 0.93；基于母亲们的数据：RMSEA = 0.055，NNFI = 0.93，CFI = 0.94）。

**父母体重水平**

由于测量父母身高体重的可行性不高，因此父母的 BMI 指数是通过其问卷中的身高、体重计算得出。问卷中填写的身高体重的有效性度已经得到了验证（Bolton-Smith, et al., 2000; Wada, et al., 2005）。

**父母自我报告的教养子女行为**

采用 17 项的李克特五点量表，这一问卷是在原有前人研究基础上进行修改和翻译得出的（Arredondo, et al., 2006; O'Connor, et al., 2010），用于评价父母对子女的教养子女的行为。这一量表包括以下子项目"饮食和身体活动的监管"（MO），"把食物或静坐少动行为当作奖励"（UR），"鼓励或强迫子女饮食"（PE），"限制不健康饮食和静坐少动行为"（RA）和"对子女健康饮食和身体活动的鼓励"（RF）。李克特五点量表提供可能的选项分别是：从不、极少、有时、经常、总是或者非常不同意、不同意、不确定、同意、非常同意。父母的教养子女的行为各个子项数据相加得出总分。有遗漏的数据用其他教养子女的方式的平均值代替。在父母教养子女的行为各项中最高的遗漏数据百分比为 0.9%。本研究还随机从大样本中抽取 1000

名受试者数据对问卷的结构效度进行了验证。本研究选用 LIS-REL 8.51 版统计软件进行实证的因子分析，关于该问卷的结构效度和重测信度结果请参考第三章中的表 3.3 和表 3.6。

**其他信息**

其他背景信息，比如父母教育程度、父母年龄以及家庭收入通过父母问卷获得。

**数理统计**

采用分层多元回归检验父母教养子女的方式是否是影响父母教养子女的行为和青少年饮食习惯、身体活动水平和体重水平关系的调节变量。回归分析的数据分析步骤参照检验调节效应的指南（Frazier, et al., 2004）。首先，计算研究变量间的相关系数，被发现与因变量相关的变量将作为模型的控制变量。在进入回归方程之前，所有的变量先进行标准化处理。分类变量将采用有效用的编码，比如，以 –1 代表男性，以 1 代表女性，以 –1 代表赣州，以 1 代表汕头等。控制变量将第一步进入回归方程，之后依次进入的变量是自变量、调节变量以及调节变量和自变量的交互效应。由于在每个模型同时检验了调节变量的多个效应，因此这些相关变量在同一批一起进入方程，以控制统计中 I 型错误的发生。根据 Frazier et al.（2004）等人的推荐，分别以父母在 API 问卷中关爱（或控制）亚量表的低分组和高分组在教养行为评分的低分（低于平均值一个标准差）和高分（高于平均值一个标准差）为点，绘出了用于预测因变量（青少年饮食习惯、身体活动水平和 Z – BMI）的回归线，此时其他变量均取值为 0。具体的数据分析过程请参见 Frazier 等人的建议（Frazier, et al., 2004）。

# 第三节　结　果

共计有 2143 名青少年和 1869 名父母参加了本次研究。受试青少年的年龄为 10 到 15 岁。表 6.1 总结了受试青少年的年龄、BMI、饮食习惯、身体活动水平、父母的教养行为和方式。

**表 6.1　研究对象的基本情况**

| 青少年性别，% | 百分比 |
| --- | --- |
| 男生 | 51.4 |
| 女生 | 48.6 |
| 父母性别，% | |
| 男性 | 40.4 |
| 女性 | 59.6 |
| | 平均值（标准差） |
| 青少年年龄 | 12.5（0.9） |
| 青少年 BMI | 18.6（2.8） |
| 青少年饮食习惯 | 39.3（5.3） |
| 青少年身体活动水平 | 5.1（2.8） |
| 父母 BMI | 22.2（3.0） |
| 父母教养子女的行为 | |
| 　饮食和身体活动的监管（MC） | 19.8（4.3） |
| 　把食物或静坐少动行为当作奖励（UR） | 5.4（1.8） |
| 　鼓励或强迫子女饮食（PE） | 9.8（2.1） |
| 　限制不健康饮食和静坐少动行为（RA） | 15.4（2.7） |

| | |
|---|---|
| 对子女健康饮食和身体活动的鼓励（RF） | 7.0（2.1） |
| 父母教养子女的方式 | |
| 关爱 | 23.9（5.6） |
| 控制 | 17.5（5.2） |

　　回归分析的结果显示，父母教养子女的行为，包括饮食和身体活动的监管、限制不健康饮食和静坐少动行为以及父母的关爱和控制都与青少年的饮食习惯有关，回归控制了青少年性别、年龄、父母性别和地域。数据分析还显示，父母教养子女的行为和方式可以解释青少年饮食习惯的方差的 10%。另有1%的方差可以由父母的关爱和 RA 的交互作用解释。此外，如图 6.1A 中的回归线所示，当父母关爱增加时，RA 与青少年饮食习惯的正相关关系被减弱了。

　　研究结果还显示，父母的关爱、控制和父母对子女饮食和身体活动的监管与青少年的身体活动相关。父母的控制与父母对子女饮食和身体活动监管的交互效应也与青少年的身体活动相关，虽然该效应仅仅解释了青少年的身体活动方差变异的1%。如图 6.1B 所示，数据显示，父母的高控制放大了青少年身体活动与父母对子女饮食和身体活动监管的关系。

　　研究数据显示三种父母教养子女的行为：父母对子女饮食和身体活动的监管，把食物或静坐少动行为当作对子女的奖励和鼓励或强迫子女饮食，与青少年的 Z－BMI 有关。但是，父母教养子女的方式中两个维度关爱和控制，均与青少年的 Z－BMI 不相关。研究数据还显示，父母的控制和父母对子女饮食和身体活动的监管的交互作用与青少年的体重水平相关，并解释了青少年 Z – BMI 方差的 1%。此外，如图 6.1C 所示，父母教养子女的方式中的控制调节了父母对子女饮食和身体活动的监管对青少年体重水平的影响。

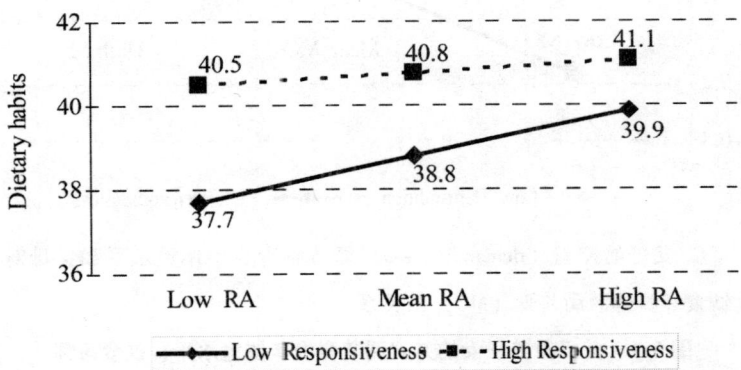

A：父母的关爱（responsiveness）调节着青少年饮食习惯与父母禁止子女不健康饮食和静坐少动行为（RA）的关系

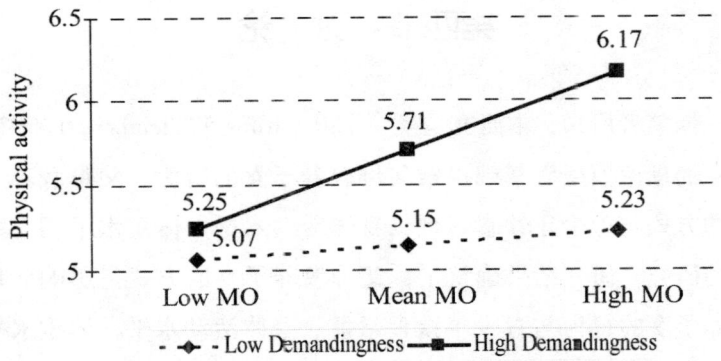

B. 父母的控制（demandingness）调节着青少年身体活动与父母对子女饮食和身体活动监管（MO）的关系

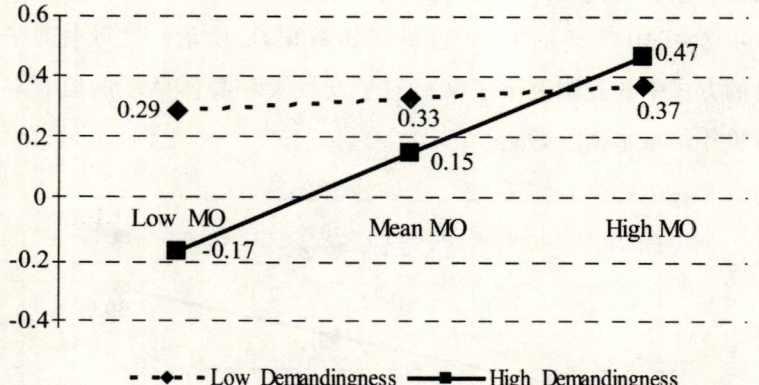

C. 父母的控制（demandingness）调节着青少年体重水平和父母对子女饮食和身体活动监管（MO）的关系

**图 6.1　父母教养子女的方式调节青少年体重水平、饮食习惯、身体活动水平与父母教养子女的行为关系的回归线**

# 第四节　讨　论

据笔者所知，本研究是第一个以 Darling 和 Steinberg（1993）建立的理论模型为基础探索父母教养子女的行为、父母教养子女的方式与青少年饮食习惯、身体活动水平、体重水平相互关系的研究。研究结果确认了，父母教养子女的方式是影响父母教养子女的行为与青少年饮食习惯、身体活动水平、体重水平关系的调节变量。

前人的研究已经报道了父母教养子女的方式对青少年饮食行为的影响。比如，有研究发现父母们控制性更强的教养子女方式往往有助于青少年少喝含糖饮料（van der Horst，Kremers，et al.，2007）。其他的研究也发现，父母采用合理而严格的教养方式有助于子女的健康饮食（Arredondo，et al.，2006）。与这些研究结果一样，本次研究也发现，父母对子女饮食和身体活动的监管、禁止子女不健康饮食和静坐少动行为以及父母的关爱和控制都与青少年的饮食健康呈正相关。此外，研究还发现，当父母对子女的关爱程度较低时，青少年的饮食行为与父母禁止子女不健康饮食和静坐少动行为的相关程度更高。这也就意味着，与对子女关爱程度高的父母抚养的青少年相比，对子女关爱程度低的父母抚养的青少年，假如父母还不控制子女摄入不健康食物的话，他们的孩子更容易出现饮食不健康的问题。相似的，本次研究的结果还发现，父母对子女的控制程度高会增强青少年身体活动水平和父母对子女饮食和身体活动监管关系。也就是说，与父母对子女控制程度低的家庭相比，在父母对子女的控制程度高的家庭中，父母对青少年身体活动的监管能够更为有效地提高青少年身体活动水平。

前期的一些研究已经证明一些父母的教养子女行为（比如对子女饮食和身体活动的监管）与青少年的体重水平有关（Faith，Berkowitz，et al.，2004）。而加强（或减少）这些与青少年体重水平相关的父母教养子女的行为的效果对于青少年肥胖的预防非常重要。而本次研究的数据表明，父母对子女的控制程度可以加强父母监管子女饮食和身体活动这一行为对青少年体重水平的影响。这一研究结果可能也部分解释了与溺爱型和放任型父母抚养的子女相比，民主型和专制型父母抚养的子女

肥胖率更低的原因 (Rhee, et al., 2006; Wake, et al., 2007)。

根据父母教养子女的方式的理论模型 (Darling & Steinberg, 1993), 父母教养子女的方式可以通过两条路径调节父母教养子女的行为与青少年的体重水平。首先，父母的教养方式可以改变父母与子女沟通的性质。比如，有研究证实，父母与子女良好的沟通有助于父母对子女的监管 (Stattin & Kerr, 2000)。因此，民主型的父母会采用更容易被子女接受的方式监管子女的饮食和身体活动，防止子女养成不良的饮食习惯和静坐少动的生活方式。第二，良好而相互尊重的父母—子女关系有助于鼓励青少年与父母交流他们的精神生活 (Stattin & Kerr, 2000)。Darling 和 Steinberg (1993) 还指出，父母的教养方式会影响青少年的个性，特别是他们对于父母教养子女的行为的接受程度，从而影响父母教养子女的行为对青少年饮食习惯、身体活动和体重水平作用的效果。

长久以来，儒家思想对中国的传统文化影响非常深远。在传统的中国家庭，父母与子女关系非常紧密，父母也是对子女生活方式影响最大的人。即使到了今天，中国社会受到了西方文明极大的影响，中国人许多教养子女的行为仍受到儒家思想的影响。中国人教养子女的方式常常被世人认为是"专制"、"严格"和"高控制"的 (Lin & Fu, 1990; Steinberg, et al., 1992)。许多基于中国父母的研究也发现，父母教养子女的方式与青少年的社会和学业表现有关 (Nelson, et al., 2006)。甚至还有研究发现，父母教养子女的方式还影响着青少年性格的形成 (Porter, et al., 2005)。而本次研究的结果进一步说明，父母教养子女的方式在青少年肥胖的发展中同样起着非常重要的作用。

表 6.2 以父母教养子女的行为、教养方式、基本信息为自变量建立的青少年体重水平、饮食习惯和身体活动水平的回归模型

| | 饮食习惯 | | | 身体活动水平 | | | 身体活动水平 | | |
| --- | --- | --- | --- | --- | --- | --- | --- | --- | --- |
| | B | 95%CI | ΔR² | B | 95%CI | ΔR² | Z-BMIB | 95%CI | ΔR² |
| 第一步ᵃ：控制变量 | | | 0.03 | | | 0.09 | | | 0.10 |
| 青少年性别 | 0.47** | 0.23, 0.71 | | -0.82** | -0.94, -0.69 | | -0.09 | -0.27, 0.08 | |
| 青少年年龄 | -0.57** | -0.82, -0.32 | | -0.20** | -0.33, -0.07 | | -0.29** | -0.49, -0.10 | |
| 父母性别 | 0.04 | -0.20, 0.29 | | 0.04 | -0.09, 0.17 | | -0.01 | -0.19, 0.17 | |
| 地域 | -0.67** | -1.17, -0.17 | | -0.90** | -1.17, -0.64 | | 0.04 | -0.33, 0.41 | |
| 青少年发育程度 | N | N | | N | N | | 0.45** | 0.25, 0.65 | |
| 父母的 BMI | N | N | | N | N | | 0.33** | 0.15, 0.50 | |
| 第二步：预测变量和调节变量 | | | 0.10 | | | 0.04 | | | 0.06 |
| MO | 0.64** | 0.24, 1.03 | | 0.27** | 0.08, 0.47 | | 0.18* | 0.04, 0.33 | |
| RF | -0.08 | -0.44, 0.28 | | -0.01 | -0.19, 0.16 | | 0.02 | -0.12, 0.15 | |
| UR | -0.14 | -0.52, 0.25 | | 0.00 | -0.06, 0.05 | | 0.25** | 0.11, 0.39 | |
| PE | -0.23 | -0.60, 0.15 | | Nᵇ | Nᵇ | | -0.50** | -0.64, -0.36 | |
| RA | 0.71** | 0.34, 1.09 | | 0.01 | -0.18, 0.19 | | 0.01 | -0.13, 0.15 | |

| | 饮食习惯 | | | 身体活动水平 | | | 身体活动水平 | | |
|---|---|---|---|---|---|---|---|---|---|
| | B | 95%CI | $\Delta R^2$ | B | 95%CI | $\Delta R^2$ | Z－BMIB | 95%CI | $\Delta R^2$ |
| 关爱 | 0.95** | 0.62, 1.28 | | 0.27** | 0.09, 0.44 | | 0.00 | -0.12, 0.12 | |
| 控制 | 0.44* | 0.08, 0.79 | | 0.28** | 0.12, 0.44 | | -0.09 | -0.22, 0.05 | |
| 第三步[a]：预测变量×调节变量 | | | 0.01 | | | 0.01 | | | 0.01 |
| RA×关爱 | -0.43* | -0.77, -0.08 | | N | N | | N | N | |
| MO×控制 | N | N | | 0.19* | 0.00, 0.39 | | 0.14* | 0.00, 0.28 | |
| 第四步[a]：控制变量×其他变量 | | | 0.01 | | | 0.02 | | | 0.03 |
| 青少年性别×RF | N | N | | 0.18* | 0.00, 0.37 | | N | N | |
| 青少年年龄×控制 | N | N | | -0.18* | -0.35, -0.01 | | N | N | |
| 青少年年龄×RA | N | N | | N | N | | -0.20** | -0.34, -0.05 | |
| 青少年性别×PE | N | N | | N | N | | -0.17* | -0.31, -0.03 | |
| 青少年性别×关爱 | N | N | | N | N | | -0.12* | -0.24, 0.00 | |

备注：所有控制变量、预测变量和调节变量先进行标准化处理，再进行回归分析。[a]：所有的预测变量：所有的预测变量、控制变量、调节变量×其他变量都进行了测试，但是此表中仅列出了具有统计学意义的效应。[b]：PE（鼓励或强迫子女饮食）未进入青少年身体活动的预测模型；N：该变量最终未进入方程。

116

本次研究不可避免地存在一些不足，在解读研究结果时值得注意。首先，我国幅员辽阔，各地区、各民族父母教养子女的方式不尽相同。本次研究仅仅是以我国南方两个中小城市的青少年及其父母为例，探讨父母教养子女的方式对于孩子身体活动水平的影响。研究结果是否与我国其他地区一致尚需更多相关研究证实。其他可能存在不足之处还包括数据来自于受试对象的主观报告而非客观测试，研究设计为横断面调查而不是纵向跟踪研究等。尽管存在一些不足，本研究仍然成功地证明了，父母教养子女的方式是影响青少年饮食习惯、身体活动水平与父母教养子女的行为之间关系的重要调节变量。本研究强调了，父母教养子女的方式对青少年体重水平的间接影响。研究结果也提示，在青少年肥胖的干预中考虑父母教养子女的方式问题，有助于提高父母教养子女的行为的干预效果。

# 第七章　总结与讨论

在过去的 20 年中，在中国，特别是中国的城市地区，青少年的肥胖问题正日益成为严重的公共问题（Luo & Hu, 2002）。要预防青少年肥胖，那么最重要的步骤之一是确定可能与儿童肥胖发展相关的各种因素。目前的研究表明，父母在青少年肥胖的病因和治疗中也许起着重要的作用（Dietz & Robinson, 2005; Robinson, 1999）。本次研究的目的就是确定父母教养子女的行为、父母教养子女的方式、父母对子女体重的认知与青少年体重水平之间的关系。

为了完成这个目标，我们的研究分为两步进行。第一步，验证了调查问卷的有效性和可靠性，该调查问卷可以用于测量父母教养子女的行为、父母教养子女的方式以及父母对子女体重的认知。本研究已经成功地证明了，调查问卷的内容效度、结构效度、重测信度以及内部一致性是可接受的，并且证明了调查问卷适用于我国南方的青少年和他们的父母。第二步，开展了一项横断面调查，调查了中国父母教养子女的行为、父母教养子女的方式、父母对子女体重的认知与青少年饮食习惯、身体活动水平、体重情况的相互关系。研究发现，青少年体重状况、饮食习惯和体育活动与某些父母教养子女的行为存在较弱的相关，但仍具有统计学意义。这些父母教养子女的行为包括：鼓励或强迫子女饮食、限制子女不健康饮食和静坐少动行为、对子女饮食和身体活动的监管等。另外，研究发现父母对子女体重的认知除了和父母的性别，子女性别以及子女对自己体重的认知相联系，还可能和一些与青少年肥胖的发展有关的父母教养子女的行为有关。此外，研究也发现，青少年的饮食习惯、身体活动以及一些父母教养子女的行为和方式密切相关。然而，我们并未发现父母教养子女的方式和青少年体重水平的直接联系。几个和父母相关的因素，包括遗传因素、家庭环境和社区建设环境及安全等方面的因素，在目前的研究中没有调查。研究提出的理论模型或许不能全面地概括所有父母相关的因素与青少年体重状况之间的关系。然而，这项研究中的发现可以帮助我们更好地理解，在中国，父母教养子女的行为和方式、父母对孩子体重的认知与青少年超重问题之间的内在关系，这对于了解我国青少年肥胖的病因、发展和治疗是非常重要的。

考虑到中国的社会环境和传统文化不同于西方国家，我们假定中国父母对孩子体重的影响会与美国和欧洲父母的情况有所不同。然而，本次研究揭示的大部分结果与西方国家报道的调查结果一致。例如，虽然青少年肥胖症的发病率仍然低于发达国家（Ji & Working Group on Obesity in China, 2005），但是在这项研究中，中国的父母们并没有展现出比欧美国家父母更好的分辨儿童体重水平的能力。此外，在传统的中国文化中，父亲与母亲在教育子女中扮演着不同的角色（Berndt，et al.，1993）。然而，我们假设的父母教养子女行为的性别差异在本次研究中并未被发现。过去几十年我国社会的变迁和西方文化的影响也许能够在一定程度上解释这一结果。

在过去几年中，关于父母参与儿童肥胖治疗的研究引起了许多研究者的注意。一些学者甚至推动了单独针对父母的干预方案，在这种干预方案中，只有父母（而不是青少年）被作为干预的目标（Golan & Weizman，2001）。一些研究已经证明了该种干预方式的有效性（Golan & Crow，2004b；McGarvey，et al.，2004）。然而，一些其他的研究数据则表明：父母对子女的教养行为也许只能解释相对较低比例的青少年食物摄入量（O'Connor，et al.，2010）和身体活动的变化（Davison，et al.，2003）。本次研究的数据也证实了父母教养子女的行为、父母教养子女的方式、父母对子女体重的认知与青少年肥胖发展之间的相互联系。虽然变量间的相关性不大，但是仍具有统计学意义。我们的研究数据支持其他学者提出的将父母的参与纳入青少年的肥胖干预治疗的观点（Dietz & Robinson，2005；Robinson，1999）。然而，由于与父母有关的因素只能解释青少年 Z-BMI、饮食习惯和肢体活动的较低比例，我们认为父母在青少年肥胖症的成因、发展和治疗中只能起重要的辅助作用而非决定作用。

现在大部分的肥胖家庭研究都集中于父母对孩子饮食习惯、身体锻炼和体重水平的影响（Anderssen & Wold，1992；Heinberg，et al.，2009；Moore，et al.，1991；Savage，et al.，2007；Wrotniak，et al.，2004）。实际上，父母和子女之间的关系可能

是双向的。例如，有研究发现，子女在帮助他们的父母戒烟上起着重要作用（Winickoff, et al. , 2006）。因此，子女也可能可以帮助他们的父母矫正饮食习惯和增加身体活动，这种理念也可以应用于成年人的健康促进中。由于本次研究采用的是横断面调查的研究设计，还无法确定其中变量的因果关系。因此，仍需要开展更多的研究来进一步探索父母在子女肥胖的发展中扮演的角色以及子女对父母行为的影响。

另一方面，当父母参与到青少年肥胖的干预治疗中时，还应该考虑到父母与子女的矛盾冲突。一项基于中国青少年和他们父母的研究显示，青少年希望获得比父母准许的更多的自主权（Yau & Smetana, 1996）。在中国大陆的一项研究中，发现有饮食障碍的年轻人与父母存在 3 种冲突类型：1. 两代间控制权和自主权的冲突；2. 长大成人和保持童真的冲突；3. 追求个人目标和不辜负父母的期望间的冲突。（J. L. C. Ma, 2008）由于在父母参与的儿童肥胖干预方案中，父母需要帮助子女改掉静坐少动行为和不健康的饮食习惯，可以预见青少年和他们的父母之间的冲突的可能会有所增加，这也可能会极大地影响干预的有效性。所以，建议在干预的过程中，应妥善处理父母和子女的关系，并应该向父母提供教育子女技巧的相关培训。

虽然目前研究的结果支持家长可能在青少年肥胖的发展中起重要作用，但一些其他的因素，比如同伴和学校的影响，在儿童肥胖的干预中的作用也应被考虑。和谐的同伴关系不仅为儿童在认知、心理和情感的发展上提供重要的环境，而且还会影响孩子的身体活动、饮食习惯和体重水平（Salvy, et al. , 2008；

Salvy，et al.，2009；Storch，et al.，2007）。例如，有研究发现，孩子们在亲密的朋友陪伴下会参与更多剧烈的身体活动（Salvy，et al.，2008）。此外，学校也可以通过体育课的多少和体育活动的强度（The National Institute of Child Health Human Development Study of Early Child Care and Youth Development Network，2003）以及在学校出售的饮料和食品（Committee on School Health，2004）来影响儿童的体重水平。因此，要将对青少年肥胖干预的效果最大化，就应该考虑到包括父母、同伴、学校等所有相关因素。

这本书的不足可能包括横向调查的研究设计、自我报告式的数据，以及不具有国家代表性的抽样样本。因此，在本次研究中，无法确定变量之间的因果的关系，研究结果可能也并不适用于世界各地的华人。我们建议在未来的研究中采用纵向跟踪的研究设计并采用客观的实验仪器进行数据收集（比如，采用加速器来测量青少年的身体活动水平等）。

综上所述，本次研究数据表明，本次研究所采用的问卷具有良好的可靠性和有效性。父母对子女的教养行为与青少年肥胖存在弱相关，但相关具有统计学意义。在中国，父母常常不能正确认识子女的体重水平，而且父母们对子女肥胖的认知与他们所采用的一些可能影响子女体重水平的教养子女的行为是相关的。此外，研究还发现，父母教养子女的方式可以调节父母教养子女行为与青少年饮食习惯、身体活动、体重水平的关系。

# 参考资料

Aaron, D. J., Kriska, A. M., Dearwater, S. R., Anderson, R. L., Olsen, T. L., Cauley, J. A., et al. (1993). The epidemiology of leisure physical activity in an adolescent population. *Medicine & Science in Sports & Exercise*, 25 (7), 847 – 853.

Adams, E. J., Grummer-Strawn, L., & Chavez, G. (2003). Food insecurity is associated with increased risk of obesity in California women. *Journal of Nutrition Education*, 133 (4), 1070 – 1074.

Addessi, E., Galloway, A. T., Visalberghi, E., & Birch, L. L. (2005). Specific social influences on the acceptance of novel foods in 2 – 5 – year – old children. *Appetite*, 45 (3), 264 – 271.

Adkins, S., Sherwood, N. E., Story, M., & Davis, M. (2004). Physical activity among African-American girls: The role of parents and the home environment. *Obesity Research*, 12 (S9), 38S – 45S.

Altabe, M. (1998). Ethnicity and body image: quantitative and qualitative analysis. *International Journal of Eating Disorders*, 23 (2), 153 – 159.

Anderssen, N. , & Wold, B. (1992). Parental and peer influences on leisure-time physical activity in young adolescents. *Research Quarterly for Exercise and Sport*, 63 (4), 341 –348.

Anguita, R. M. , Sigulem, D. M. , & Sawaya, A. L. ( 1993 ). Intrauterine food restriction is associated with obesity in young rats. *Journal of Nutrition Education*, 123 (8), 1421 –1428.

Arredondo, E. M. , Elder, J. P. , Ayala, G. X. , Campbell, N. , Baquero, B. , & Duerksen, S. (2006). Is parenting style related to children's healthy eating and physical activity in Latino families? *Health Education Research*, 21 (6), 862 –871.

Aunola, K. , Stattin, H. , & Nurmi, J. E. (2000). Parenting styles and adolescents' achievement strategies. *Journal of Adolescence*, 23 (2), 205 –222.

Ball, K. , & Crawford, D. (2005a). The role of socio-cultural factors in the obesity epidemic. In D. Crawford & R. W. Jeffery ( Eds. ), *Obesity prevention and public health* ( pp. 37 – 53 ). New York: Oxford University Press.

Ball, K. , & Crawford, D. (2005b). Socioeconomic status and weight change in adults: a review. *Social Science & Medicine*, 60 (9), 1987 –2010.

Ball, K. , Mishra, G. D. , & Crawford, D. ( 2003 ). Social factors and obesity: an investigation of the role of health behaviours. *International Journal of Obesity*, 27 (3), 394 –403.

Bandini, L. G. , Must, A. , Spadano, J. L. , & Dietz, W. H.

(2002). Relation of body composition, parental overweight, pubertal stage, and race-ethnicity to energy expenditure among premenarcheal girls. *American Journal of Clinical Nutrition*, 76 (5), 1040 – 1047.

Banville, D. , Desrosiers, P. , & Ganet-Volet, Y. ( 2000 ). Translating questionnaires and inventories using a cross-cultural translation technique. *Journal of Teaching in Physical Education*, 19, 374 – 387.

Barlow, S. E. , & the Expert Committee (2007). Expert committee recommendations regarding the prevention, assessment, and treatment of child and adolescent overweight and obesity: Summary report. . *Pediatrics*, 120 (Supplement 4), S164 – 192.

Batsell, W. R. , Brown, A. S. , Ansfield, M. E. , & Paschall, G. Y. ( 2002 ). "You will eat all of that!": A retrospective analysis of forced consumption episodes. *Appetite*, 38 (3), 211 – 219.

Baughcum, A. E. , Burklow, K. A. , Deeks, C. M. , Powers, S. W. , & Whitaker, R. C. ( 1998 ). Maternal feeding practices and childhood obesity: A focus group study of low-income mothers. *Archives of Pediatrics & Adolescent Medicine*, 152 (10), 1010 – 1014.

Baughcum, A. E. , Chamberlin, L. A. , Deeks, C. M. , Powers, S. W. , & Whitaker, R. C. (2000). Maternal perceptions of overweight preschool children. *Pediatrics*, 106 (6), 1380 – 1386.

Baumgartner, T. A. , & Jackson, A. S. ( 1996 ). *Measurement for evaluation in physical education and exercise science* ( 6th ed. ). Boston, MA: WCB McGraw-Hill.

Baumgartner, T. A. , & Jackson, A. S. (1999). *Measurement for evaluation in physical education and exercise science* (6th ed. ). Boston, MA: WCB McGraw-Hill.

Baumrind, D. (1971). Current patterns of parental authority. *Developmental Psychology*, 4 (1, Part 2), 1 – 103.

Baumrind, D. (1991). The influence of parenting style on adolescent competence and substance use. *The Journal of Early Adolescence*, 11 (1), 56 – 95.

Berndt, T. J. , Cheung, P. C. , Lau, S. , Hau, K. – T. , & Lew, W. J. F. (1993). Perceptions of parenting in mainland China, Taiwan, and Hong Kong: Sex differences and societal differences *Developmental Psychology*, 29 (1), 156 – 164.

Beunen, G. , Maes, H. H. , Vlietinck, R. , Malina, R. M. , Thomis, M. , Feys, E. , et al. (1998). Univariate and multivariate genetic analysis of subcutaneous fatness and fat distribution in early adolescence. *Behavior Genetics*, 28 (4), 279.

Birch, L. L. , & Fisher, J. O. (1998). Development of eating behaviors among children and adolescents. *Pediatrics*, 101 (3), 539 – 549.

Birch, L. L. , Fisher, J. O. , Grimm-Thomas, K. , Markey, C. N. , Sawyer, R. , & Johnson, S. L. (2001). Confirmatory factor analysis of the Child Feeding Questionnaire: a measure of parental attitudes, beliefs and practices about child feeding and obesity proneness. *Appetite*, 36 (3), 201 – 210.

Birch, L. L. , Zimmerman, S. I. , & Hind, H. (1980). The influence of social-affective context on the formation of children's food preferences. *Child Development*, 51 (3), 856 – 861.

Bittner Fagan, H. , Diamond, J. , Myers, R. , & Gill, J. M. (2008). Perception, intention, and action in adolescent obesity. *The Journal of the American Board of Family Medicine*, 21 (6), 555 – 561.

Blanchette, L , & Brug, J. (2005). Determinants of fruit and vegetable consumption among 6 – 12 – year – old children and effective interventions to increase consumption. *Journal of Human Nutrition and Dietetics*, 18 (6), 431 – 443.

Bogardus, C. , Lillicja, S. , Ravussin, E. , Abbott, W. , Zawadzki, J. K. , Young, A. , et al. (1986). Familial dependence of the resting metabolic rate. *The New England Journal of Medicine*, 315 (2), 96 – 100.

Bolton-Smith, C. , Woodward, M. , Tunstall-Pedoe, H. , & Morrison, C. (2000). Accuracy of the estimated prevalence of obesity from self reported height and weight in an adult Scottish population. *Journal of Epidemiology and Community Health*, 54 (2), 143 – 148.

Bond, M. H. , & Hwang, K. K. (1986). The social psychology of Chinese people. In M. H. Bond (Ed.), *The psychology of the Chinese people* (pp. 213 – 264). Hong Kong: Oxford University Press.

Bosy-Westphal, A. , Wolf, A. , Buhrens, F , Hitze, B. , Czech, N. , Monig, H. , et al. (2008). Familial influences and obesity-associated metabolic risk factors contribute to the variation in resting energy expenditure: The Kiel obesity prevention study. *American Journal of Clinical Nutrition*, 87 (6), 1695 – 1701.

Bouchard, C. , Tremblay, A. , Nadeau, A. , Despres, J. P. , Theriault, G. , Boulay, M. R. , et al. ( 1989 ). Genetic effect in resting and exercise metabolic rates. *Metabolism*, 38 (4), 364 – 370.

Bourcier, E. , Bowen, D. J. , Meischke, H. , & Moinpour, C. (2003). Evaluation of strategies used by family food preparers to influence healthy eating. *Appetite*, 41 (3), 265 – 272.

Bowman, S. A. , Gortmaker, S. L. , Ebbeling, C. B. , Pereira, M. A. , & Ludwig, D. S. (2004). Effects of fast-food consumption on energy intake and diet quality among children in a national household survey. *Pediatrics*, 113 (1), 112 – 118.

Bulik, C. M. , Sullivan, P. F. , & Kendler, K. S. ( 2003 ). Genetic and environmental contributions to obesity and binge eating. *International Journal of Eating Disorders*, 33 (3), 293 – 298.

Burdette, H. L. , & Whitaker, R. C. ( 2004 ). Neighborhood playgrounds, fast food restaurants, and crime: relationships to overweight in low-income preschool children. *Preventive Medicine*, 38 (1), 57 – 63.

Burdette, H. L. , & Whitaker, R. C. (2005). A national study of neighborhood safety, outdoor play, television viewing, and obesity in preschool children. *Pediatrics*, 116 (3), 657 – 662.

Butte, N. F. , Garza, C. , & de Onis, M. (2007). Evaluation of the feasibility of international growth standards for school-aged children and adolescents. *The Journal of Nutrition*, 137 (1), 153 – 157.

Campbell, M. W. , Williams, J. , Hampton, A. , & Wake, M. ( 2006 ). Maternal concern and perceptions of overweight in Australian preschool-aged children. *The Medical Journal of Australia*, 184, 274 – 277.

Chan, N. P. , Sung, R. Y. T. , Kong, A. P. S. , Goggins, W. B. , So, H. K. , & Nelson, E. A. S. ( 2008 ). Reliability of pubertal self-assessment in Hong Kong Chinese children. *Journal of Pediatrics and Child Health*, 44 (6), 353 – 358.

Chao, R. K. (1994). Beyond parental control and authoritarian parenting style: Understanding Chinese parenting through the cultural notion of training. *Child Development*, 65 (4), 1111 – 1119

Chen, B. , Li, H. F. , Wang, G. J. , Liu, Y. X. , Lei, Y. , & Li, S. L. (2008). Epidemiologtical study on obesity of children aged 0 – 6 years in Shenzhen. *Chinese Journal of Child Health Care*, 16 (6), 692 – 694.

Chen, F. M. , & Luster, T. (2002). Factors related to parenting practices in Taiwan. *Early Child Development and Care*, 172 (5), 413 – 430.

Chen, J. L. , & Kennedy, C. (2004). Family functioning, parenting style, and Chinese children's weight status. *Journal of Family Nursing*, 10 (2), 262 – 279.

Chen, X. Y. , Dong, Q. , & Zhou, H. (1997). Authoritative and authoritarian parenting practices and social and school performance in

Chinese children. *International Journal of Behavioral Development*, 21 (4), 855 – 873.

Choquet, M. , Hassler, C. , Morin, D. , Falissard, B. , & Chau, N. (2008). Perceived parenting styles and tobacco, alcohol and cannabis use among french adolescents: Gender and family structure differentials. *Alcohol and Alcoholism* 43 (1), 73 – 80.

Choudhary, A. K. , Donnelly, L. F. , Racadio, J. M. , & Strife, J. L. (2007). Diseases associated with childhood obesity. *American Journal of Roentgenology*, 188 (4), 1118 – 1130.

Clark, H. R. , Goyder, E. , Bissell, P. , Blank, L. , & Peters, J. (2007). How do parents' child-feeding behaviours influence child weight? Implications for childhood obesity policy. *Journal of Public Health*, 29 (2), 132 – 141.

Collins, M. E. (1991). Body figure perceptions and preferences among preadolescent children. *International Journal of Eating Disorders*, 10 (2), 199 – 208.

Committee on School Health (2004). Soft drinks in schools. *Pediatrics*, 113 (1), 152 – 154.

Cullen, K. W. , Baranowski, T. , Owens, E. , Marsh, T. , Rittenberry, L. , & de Moor, C. (2003). Availability, accessibility, and preferences for fruit, 100% fruit juice, and vegetables influence children's dietary behavior. *Health Education & Behavior*, 30 (5), 615 – 626.

Dabelea, D. , Mayer-Davis, E. J. , Lamichhane, A. P. ,

D'Agostino, R. B. , Jr. , Liese, A. D. , Vehik, K. S. , et al. ( 2008 ). Association of intrauterine exposure to maternal diabetes and obesity with type 2 diabetes in youth: the SEARCH case-control study. *Diabetes Care*, 31 (7), 1422 – 1426.

Danner, F. W. ( 2008 ). A national longitudinal study of the association between hours of TV viewing and the trajectory of BMI growth among US children. *Journal of Pediatric Psychology*, 33 (10), 1100 – 1107.

Darling, N. , & Steinberg, L. ( 1993 ). Parenting style as context: An integrative model. *Psychological Bulletin*, 113 (3), 487 – 496.

Davies, P. S. , Wells, J. C. , Fieldhouse, C. A. , Day, J. M. , & Lucas, A. (1995). Parental body composition and infant energy expenditure. *American Journal of Clinical Nutrition*, 61 (5), 1026 – 1029.

Davison, K. K. , Cutting, T. M. , & Birch, L. L. ( 2003 ). Parents' activity-related parenting practices predict girls' physical activity. *Medicine & Science in Sports & Exercise*, 35 (9), 1589 – 1595.

De Onis, M. , Onyango, A. W. , Borghi, E. , Siyam, A. , Nishida, C. , & Siekmann, J. ( 2007 ). Development of a WHO growth reference for school-aged children and adolescents. *Bulletin of the World Health Organization*, 85 (9), 660 – 667.

Deutsch, F. M. (2006). Filial piety, patrilineality, and China's one-child policy. *Journal of Family Issues*, 27 (3), 366 – 389.

Dietz, W. H. ( 1994 ). Critical periods in childhood for the development of obesity. *American Journal of Clinical Nutrition*, 59 (5), 955 – 959.

Dietz, W. H., & Robinson, T. N. (2005). Overweight children and adolescents. *The New England Journal of Medicine*, 352 (20), 2100 – 2109.

Dunton, G. F., Jamner, M. S., & Cooper, D. M. (2003). Assessing the perceived environment among minimally active adolescent girls: validity and relations to physical activity outcomes. *American Journal of Health Promotion*, 18 (1), 70 – 73.

Eckstein, K. C., Mikhail, L. M., Ariza, A. J., Thomson, J. S., Millard, S. C., Binns, H. J., et al. (2006). Parents' perceptions of their child's weight and health. *Pediatrics*, 117 (3), 681 – 690.

Elder, J. P., Ayala, G. X., & Harris, S. (1999). Theories and intervention approaches to health-behavior change in primary care. *American Journal of Preventive Medicine*, 17 (4), 275.

Epstein, L. H., Valoski, A., Wing, R. R., & McCurley, J. (1990). Ten-year follow-up of behavioral, family-based treatment for obese children. *The Journal f American Medical Association*, 264 (19), 2519 – 2523.

Etelson, D., Brand, D. A., Patrick, P. A., & Shirali, A. (2003). Childhood obesity: Do parents recognize this health risk? *Obesity Research* 11, 1362 – 1368.

Fabsitz, R. R., Sholinsky, P., & Carmelli, D. (1994).

Genetic influences on adult weight gain and maximum body mass index in male twins. *American Journal of Epidemiology*, 140 (8), 711 – 720.

Faith, M. S. , Berkowitz, R. I. , Stallings, V. A. , Kerns, J. , Storey, M. , & Stunkard. A. J. (2004). Parental feeding attitudes and styles and child body mass index: prospective analysis of a gene-environment interaction. *Pediatrics*, 114 (4), e429 – 436.

Faith, M. S. , Pietrobelli, A. , Nunez, C. , Heo, M. , Heymsfield, S. B. , & Allison, D. B. (1999). Evidence for independent genetic influences on fat mass and body mass index in a pediatric twin sample. *Pediatrics*, 104 (1), 61 – 67.

Faith, M. S. , Rhea, S. A. , Corley, R. P. , & Hewitt, J. K. (2008). Genetic and shared environmental influences on children's 24 – h food and beverage intake: sex differences at age 7 y. *American Journal of Clinical Nutrition*, 87 (4), 903 – 911.

Faith, M. S. , Scanlon, K. S. , Birch, L. L. , Francis, L. A. , & Sherry, B. (2004). Parent – child feeding strategies and their relationships to child eating and weight status. *Obesity Research*, 12 (11), 1711 – 1722.

Figueroa – Colon, R. , Arani, R. B. , Goran, M. I. , & Weinsier, R. L. (2000). Paternal body fat is a longitudinal predictor of changes in body fat in premenarcheal girls. *American Journal of Clinical Nutrition*, 71 (3), 829 – 834.

Fisher, J. C. , & Birch, L. L. (1999a). Restricting access to foods and children's eating. *Appetite*, 32 (3), 405 – 419.

Fisher, J. O. , & Birch, L. L. (1999b). Restricting access to palatable foods affects children's behavioral response, food selection, and intake. *American Journal of Clinical Nutrition*, 69 (6), 1264 – 1272.

Fisher, J. O. , & Birch, L. L. (2002). Eating in the absence of hunger and overweight in girls from 5 to 7 y of age. *American Journal of Clinical Nutrition*, 76 (1), 226 – 231.

Fisher, J. O. , Mitchell, D. C. , Wright, H. S. , & Birch, L. L. (2002). Parental influences on young girls' fruit and vegetable, micronutrient, and fat intakes. *Journal of the American Dietetic Association*, 102 (1), 58 – 64.

Fitgerald, J. T. , Singleton, S. P. , Neale, A. V. , Prasad, A. S. , & Hess, J. W. (1994). Activity levels, fitness status, exercise knowledge, and exercise beliefs among healthy, older African American and white women. *Journal of Aging Health*, 6 (3), 296 – 313.

Fonseca, H. , & Gaspar de Matos, M. (2005). Perception of overweight and obesity among Portuguese adolescents: an overview of associated factors. *The European Journal of Public Health*, 15 (3), 323 – 328.

Foster, G. D. , Sherman, S. , Borradaile, K. E. , Grundy, K. M. , Vander Veur, S. S. , Nachmani, J. , et al. (2008). A Policy-based school intervention to prevent overweight and obesity.

*Pediatrics*, 121 (4), e794 –802.

Franzini, L. , Elliott, M. N. , Cuccaro, P. , Schuster, M. , Gilliland, M. J. , Grunbaum, J. A. , et al. ( 2009 ). Influences of physical and social neighborhood environments on children's physical activity and obesity. *American Journal of Public Health*, 99 ( 2 ), 271 –278.

Frazier, P. A. , Tix, A. P. , & Barron, K. E. ( 2004 ). Testing Moderator and Mediator Effects in Counseling Psychology Research. *Journal of Counseling Psychology*, 51 ( 1 ), 115 –134.

Ganzhou municipal bureau of statistics ( 2010 ). *Statistical communique of Ganzhou on the 2009 national economic and social development.* Ganzhou, China: Ganzhou municipal bureau of statistics.

George, J. D. , Stone, W. J. , & Burkett, L. N. ( 1997 ). Non-exercise VO2max estimation for physically active college students. *Medicine & Science in Sports & Exercise*, 29 ( 3 ), 415 –423.

Gibson, E. L. , Wardle, J. , & Watts, C. J. ( 1998 ). Fruit and vegetable consumption, nutritional knowledge and beliefs in mothers and children. *Appetite*, 31 ( 2 ), 205 –228.

Gluck, M. E. , & Geliebter, A. ( 2002 ). Racial/ethnic differences in body image and eating behaviors. *Eating Behaviors*, 3 ( 2 ), 143 –151.

Godin, G. , & Shephard, R. J. ( 1985 ). A simple method to assess exercise behavior in the community. *Canadian Journal of Applied Sport Sciences*, 10 ( 3 ), 141 –146.

Golan, M. , & Crow, S. ( 2004a ). Parents are key players in the prevention and treatment of weight-related problems. *Nutrition Review*, 62 ( 1 ), 39 – 50.

Golan, M. , & Crow, S. ( 2004b ). Targeting parents exclusively in the treatment of childhood obesity: long-term results. *Obesity Research* 12 ( 2 ), 357 – 361.

Golan, M. , & Weizman, A. ( 1998 ). Reliability and validity of the Family Eating and Activity Habits Questionnaire. *European Journal of Clinical Nutrition*, 52 ( 10 ), 771 – 777.

Golan, M. , & Weizman, A. ( 2001 ). Familial approach to the treatment of childhood obesity: conceptual model. *Journal of Nutrition Education*, 33 ( 2 ), 102 – 107.

Goran, M. I. ( 2001 ). Metabolic precursors and effects of obesity in children: a decade of progress, 1990 – 1999. *American Journal of Clinical Nutrition*, 73 ( 2 ), 158 – 171.

Goran, M. I. , Carpenter, W. H. , McGloin, A. , Johnson, R. , Hardin, J. M. , & Weinsier, R. L. ( 1995 ). Energy expenditure in children of lean and obese parents. *American Journal of Physiology-Endocrinology and Metabolism*, 268 ( 5 ), E917 – 924.

Gordon-Larsen, P. ( 2001 ). Obesity-related knowledge, attitudes, and behaviors in obese and non-obese urban Philadelphia female adolescents. *Obesity*, 9 ( 2 ), 112 – 118.

Griffiths, M. , & Payne, P. R. ( 1976 ). Energy expenditure in small children of obese and non-obese parents. *Nature*, 260

(5553), 698 – 700.

Griffiths, M. , Payne, P. R. , Stunkard, A. J. , Rivers, J. P. W. , & Cox, M. (1990). Metabolic rate and physical development in children at risk of obesity. *Lancet*, 336 (8707), 76 –78.

Grimmett, C. , Croker, H. , Carnell, S. , & Wardle, J. (2008). Telling parents their child's weight status: psychological impact of a weight-screening program. *Pediatrics*, 122 (3), e682 –688.

Gunnell, D. J. , Frankel, S. J. , Nanchahal, K. , Peters, T. J. , & Davey Smith, G. (1998). Childhood obesity and adult cardiovascular mortality: a 57-y follow-up study based on the Boyd Orr cohort. *American Journal of Clinical Nutrition*, 67 (6), 1111 – 1118.

Ha, A. S. , Macdonald, D. , & Pang, B. O. (2010). Physical activity in the lives of Hong Kong Chinese children. *Sport*, *Education and Society*, 15 (3), 331 – 346.

Hagger, M. S. , Chatzisarantis, N. L. D. , & Biddle, S. J. H. (2002). Ameta-analytic review of the theories of reasoned action and planned behavior in physical activity: predictive validity and the contribution of additional variables. *Journal of Sport & Exercise Psychology*, 24 (1), 3 –32.

Harrell, J. S. , Bomar, P. , McMurray, R. , Bradley, C. , & Deng, S. (2001). Leptin and obesity in mother-child pairs. *Biological Research for Nursing*, 3 (2), 55 –64.

Hearn, M. D. , Baranowski, T. , Baranowski, J. , Doyle, C. , Smith, M. , Lin, L. S. , et al. (1998). Environmental influences on dietary behavior among children: Availability and accessibility of fruit and vegetable enable consumption. *Journal of Health Education*, 29, 26 – 32.

Heber, D. (2010). An integrative view of obesity. *The American Journal of Clinical Nutrition*, 91 (1), 280S – 283S.

Heinberg, L. J., Kutchman, E. M., Lawhun, S. A., Berger, N. A., Seabrook, R. C., Cuttler, L., et al. (2009). Parent involvement is associated with early success in obesity treatment. *Clinical Pediatrics*, published ahead-of-print.

Heitmann, B. L., Harris, J. R., Lissner, L., & Pedersen, N. L. (1999). Genetic effects on weight change and food intake in Swedish adult twins. *American Journal of Clinical Nutrition*, 69 (4), 597 – 602.

Hoddinott, P., Tappin, D., & Wright, C. (2008). Breast feeding. *British Medical Journal*, 336 (7649), 881 – 887.

Hodges, E. A. (2003). A Primer on Early Childhood Obesity and Parental Influence. *Pediatric Nursing*, 29 (1), 13 – 16.

Holroyd, E. E. (2003). Chinese cultural influences on parental caregiving obligations toward children with disabilities. *Qualitative Health Research*, 13 (1), 4 – 19.

Hooper, D., Coughlan, J., & Mullen, M. R. (2008). Structural equation modelling: Guidelines for determining model fit. *The Electronic Journal of Business Research Methods* 6 (1), 53 – 60.

Hopkins, W. G. (2000). Measures of reliability in sports medicine and science *Sports Medicine*, 30 (1), 1 – 15.

Hopper, J. L. , Bishop, D. T. , & Easton, D. F. (2005). Population-based family studies in genetic epidemiology. *Lancet*, 366, 1397 – 1406.

Howard, K. R. (2007). Childhood overweight: parental perceptions and readiness for change. *The Journal of School Nursing*, 23 (2), 73 – 79.

Huang, J. S. , Becerra, K. , Oda, T. , Walker, E. , Xu, R. , Donohue, M. , et al. (2007). Parental ability to discriminate the weight status of children: Results of a survey. *Pediatrics*, 120 (1), e112 – 119.

Hughes, S. O. , O'Connor, T. M. , & Power, T. G. (2008). Parenting and children' s eating patterns: Examining control in a broader context. *International Journal of Child and Adolescent Health*, 1 (4), 323 – 330.

Hughes, S. O. , Power, T. G. , Fisher, J. O. , Mueller, S. , & Nicklas, T. A. (2003). The development of the Caregiver's Feeding Styles Questionnaire. *Journal of the American Dietetic Association*, 103 (Supplement 9), 20.

Hui, S. C. (2001). Criterion-related validity of a 0 – 10 scale physical activity rating in Chinese youth, 2001 *Asia-Pacific Rim Conference on Exercise and Sports Science: The New Perspective of Exercise & Sports Science for the Better Life in the 21st Century* (pp. 159). Seoul, Korea: Seoul National University.

Hui, S. C. , Chan, C. M. , Wong, S. H. S. , Ha, A. S. C. , & Hong, Y. (2001). Physical activity levels of Chinese youths and its association with physical fitness and demographic variables: The Hong Kong youth fitness study. *Research Quarterly for Exercise and Sport*, 72 (supplement), A72 – 73.

Jackson, C. , Henriksen, L. , & Foshee, V. A. (1998). The authoritative parenting index: Predicting health risk behaviors among children and adolescents. *Health Education & Behavior*, 25 (3), 319 – 337.

Jakicic, J. M. , & Otto, A. D. (2005). Physical activity considerations for the treatment and prevention of obesity. *American Journal of Clinical Nutrition*, 82(1), 226S – 229S.

Janz, N. K. , & Becker, M. H. (1984). The Health Belief Model: A Decade Later. *Health education quarterly*, 11 (1), 1 – 47.

Jeffery, R. W. , & French, S. A. (1996). Socioeconomic status and weight control practices among 20 – to 45 – year – old women. *American Journal of Public Health*, 86 (7), 1005 – 1010.

Jeffery, R. W. , & French, S. A. (1998). Epidemic obesity in the United States: are fast foods and television viewing contributing? *American Journal of Public Health*, 88 (2), 277 – 280.

Ji, C. Y. , & Working Group on Obesity in China (2005). Report on childhood obesity in China (1) body mass index reference for screening overweight and obesity in Chinese school-age children.

*Biomedical and Environmental Sciences*, 18 (6), 390 – 400.

Jiang, J. X. , Rosenqvist, U. , Wang, H. , Greiner, T. , Ma, Y. , & Toschke, A. M. (2006). Risk factors for overweight in 2 – to 6 – year – old children in Beijing, China. *International Journal of Pediatric Obesity* 1 (2), 103 – 108.

Jiang, J. X. , Rosenqvist, U. , Wang, H. S. , Greiner, T. , Lian, G. L. , & Sarkadi, A. (2007). Influence of grandparents on eating behaviors of young children in Chinese three-generation families. *Appetite*, 48 (3), 377 – 383.

Jing, Q. C. (1994). The Chinese single-child family programme and population psychology. *Psychology Developing Societies*, 6 (1), 29 – 52.

Kaplowitz, P. B. , Slora, E. J. , Wasserman, R. C. , Pedlow, S. E. , & Herman-Giddens, M. E. (2001). Earlier onset of puberty in girls: Relation to increased body mass index and race. *Pediatrics*, 108 (2), 347 – 353.

Kim, S. , & Douthitt, R. A. (2003). Mothers' health awareness and its impact on children's dairy product intakes. *Family and Consumer Sciences Research Journal*, 31(3), 272 – 296.

Kimiecik, J. C. , Horn, T. S. , & Shurin, C. S. (1996). Relationships among children's beliefs, perceptions of their parents' beliefs, and their moderate-to-vigorous physical activity. *Research Quarterly for Exercise and Sport*, 67 (3), 324 – 336.

King, K. A. , Tergerson, J. L. , & Wilson, B. R. (2008).

Effect of social support on adolescents' perceptions of and engagement in physical activity. *Journal of Physical Activity & Health*, 5 (3), 374 – 384.

Klesges, R. C. , Stein, R. J. , Eck, L. H. , Isbell, T. R. , & Klesges, L. M. (1991). Parental influence on food selection in young children and its relationships to childhood obesity. *American Journal of Clinical Nutrition*, 53 (4), 859 – 864.

Klohe-Lehman, D. M. , Freeland-Graves, J. , Clarke, K. K. , Cai, G. , Voruganti, V. S. , Milani, T. J. , et al. (2007). Low-income, overweight and obese mothers as agents of change to improve food choices, fat habits, and physical activity in their 1 – to – 3 – year – old children. *Journal of American College of Nutrition*, 26 (3), 196 – 208.

Koletzko, B. , von Kries, R. , Monasterolo, R. C. , Subias, J. E. , Scaglioni, S. , Giovannini, M. , et al. (2009). Can infant feeding choices modulate later obesity risk? *American Journal of Clinical Nutrition*, 89 (5), 1502S – 1508S.

Kong, A. , Choi, K. – C. , Li, A. , Hui, S. , Chan, M. , Wing, Y. , et al. (2010). Association between Physical Activity and Cardiovascular Risk in Chinese Youth Independent of Age and Pubertal Stage. *BMC Public Health*, 10 (1), 303.

Kramer, M. S. , Matush, L. , Vanilovich, I. , Platt, R. W. , Bogdanovich, N. , Sevkovskaya, Z. , et al. (2008). A randomized breast-feeding promotion intervention did not reduce child obesity in

Belarus. *The Journal of Nutrition*, 139 (2), 417S–421S.

Kroller, K. , & Warschburger, P. (2009). Maternal feeding strategies and child's food intake: considering weight and demographic influences using structural equation modeling. *International Journal of Behavioral Nutrition and Physical Activity*, 6 (1), 78–86.

Larson, N. , Neumark–Sztainer, D. , Story, M. , Wall, M. , Harnack, L. , & Eisenberg, M. E. (2007). Longitudinal predictors of fruit and vegetable intake during the transition to young adulthood. *Journal of Nutrition Education and Behavior*, 39 (4, Supplement 1), S90–S90.

Lau, P. W. C. , Lee, A. , & Ransdell, L. (2007). Parenting style and cultural influences on overweight children's attraction to physical activity. *Obesity*, 15 (9), 2293–2302.

Lee, Y. , Mitchell, D. C. , Smiciklas-Wright, H. , & Birch, L. L. (2001). Diet quality, nutrient intake, weight status, and feeding environments of girls meeting or exceeding recommendations for total dietary fat of the American Academy of Pediatrics. *Pediatrics*, 107 (6), e95.

Lehingue, Y. (1999). The European Childhood Obesity Group (ECOG) project: the European collaborative study on the prevalence of obesity in children. *American Journal of Clinical Nutrition*, 70 (1), 166S–168S.

Levin, B. E. (2000). The obesity epidemic: Metabolic imprinting on genetically susceptible neural circuits. *Obesity*, 8 (4),

342 – 347.

Li, C. L. , & Li, J. Y. (2005). Research on parents opposing their children joining school sports team training. *China Sport Science and Technology*, 41 (1), 126 – 128.

Li, M. , Dibley, M. J. , Sibbritt, D. , & Yan, H. (2006). Factors associated with adolescents' physical inactivity in Xi'an city, China. *Medicine and Science in Sports and Exercise* 38 (12), 2075 – 2085

Li, Y. , Zhai, F. , Yang, X. , Schouten, E. G. , Hu, X. , He, Y. , et al. (2007). Determinants of childhood overweight and obesity in China. *British Journal of Nutrition*, 97 (01), 210 – 215.

Li, Y. N. (2008). Social analysis on reasons of childhood obesity in China cities. *Studies in Preschool Education*, 22 (3), 37 – 40.

Lin, C. – Y. C. , & Fu, V. R. (1990). A comparison of child-rearing practices among Chinese, immigrant Chinese, and Caucasian-American parents. *Child Development*, 61 (2), 429 – 433.

Lindsay, A. C. , Sussner, K. M. , Kim, J. , & Gortmaker, S. (2006). The role of parents in preventing childhood obesity. *Future Child* 16 (1), 169 – 180.

Lissau, I. , & S? rensen, T. I. (1994). Parental neglect during childhood and increased risk of obesity in young adulthood. *The Lancet*, 343 (8893), 324 – 327.

Lobstein, T. , Baur, L. , & Uauy, R. (2004). Obesity in children and young people: a crisis in public health. *Obesity Reviews*, 5 (s1), 4 – 85.

Lumeng, J. C. , & Burke, L. M. (2006). Maternal prompts to eat, child compliance, and mother and child weight status. *The Journal of Pediatrics*, 149 (3), 330 – 335.

Luo, J. , & Hu, F. B. (2002). Time trends of obesity in pre-school children in China from 1989 to 1997. *International Journal of Obesity*, 26, 553 – 558.

Lv, S. H. , & Tian, B. C. (2007). KAP changes on children's obesity control among parents after school-based intervention. *Chinese Journal of School Health*, 28 (1), 26 – 28.

Ma, G. S. (2005). Diets practices of child or teenager and relevant influencing factors. *Chinese Journal of Health Education*, 21, 337 – 340.

Ma, J. L. C. (2008). Eating disorders, parent-child conflicts, and family therapy in Shenzhen, China. *Qualitative Health Research*, 18 (6), 803 – 810.

Ma, W. J. , Du, L. , Lin, G. Z. , Ren, Y. Q. , & Ma, G. S. (2001). Family factors influencing dietary behavior of primary and secondary school students in Guangzhou city. *Chinese Journal of Disease Control and Prevention*, 5 (2), 125 – 127.

Maes, H. H. M. , Neale, M. C. , & Eaves, L. J. (1997). Genetic and environmental factors in relative body weight and human adiposity. *Behavior Genetics*, 27 (4), 325 – 351.

Magarey, A. M. , Daniels, L. M. , Boulton, T. J. , & Cockington, R. A. (2003). Predicting obesity in early adulthood from childhood and parental obesity. [Article]. *International Journal of Obesity*, 27 (4), 505 – 513.

Malis, C. , Rasmussen, E. L. , Poulsen, P. , Petersen, I. , Christensen, K. , Beck-Nielsen, H. , et al. (2005). Total and regional fat distribution is strongly influenced by genetic factors in young and elderly twins. *Obesity*, 13 (12), 2139 – 2145.

Maynard, L. M. , Galuska, D. A. , Blanck, H. M. , & Serdula, M. K. (2003). Maternal perceptions of weight status of children. *Pediatrics*, 111 (5), 1226 – 1231.

McGarvey, E. , Keller, A. , Forrester, M. , Williams, E. , Seward, D. , & Suttle, D. E. (2004). Feasibility and benefits of a parent-focused preschool child obesity intervention. *American Journal of Public Health*, 94 (9), 1490 – 1495.

McLaren, L. (2007). Socioeconomic Status and Obesity. *Epidemiologic Reviews* 29 (1), 29 – 48.

McLean, N. , Griffin, S. , Toney, K. , & Hardeman, W. (2003). Family involvement in weight control, weight maintenance and weight-loss interventions: a systematic review of randomised trials. *International Journal of Obesity*, 27 (9), 987 – 1005.

Mendez, M. A. , Monteiro, C. A. , & Popkin, B. M. (2005). Overweight exceeds underweight among women in most developing countries. *The American Journal of Clinical Nutrition*, 81 (3), 714 – 721.

Moore, L. L. , Lombardi, D. A. , White, M. J. , Campbell,

J. L. , Oliveria, S. A. , & Ellison, R. C. ( 1991 ). Influence of parents' physical activity levels on activity levels of young children. *The Journal of Pediatrics*, 118 (2), 215 – 219.

Motl, R. W. , Dishman, R. K. , Saunders, R. P. , Dowda, M. , & Pate, R. R. ( 2007 ). Perceptions of physical and social environment variables and self-efficacy as correlates of self-reported physical activity among adolescent girls. *Journal of Pediatric Psychology*, 32 (1), 6 – 12.

Motl, R. W. , Dishman, R. K. , Ward, D. S. , Saunders, R. P. , Dowda, M. , Felton, G. , et al. (2005). Perceived physical environment and physical activity across one year among adolescent girls: self-efficacy as a possible mediator? *Journal of Adolescent Health*, 37 (5), 403 – 408.

Mulvihill, C. , Rivers, K. , & Aggleton, P. (2000). A qualitative study investigating the views of primary-age children and parents on physical activity. *Health Education Journal*, 59 (2), 166 – 179.

Must, A. , & Strauss, R. S. ( 1999 ). Risks and consequences of childhood and adolescent obesity. *International Journal of Obesity*, 23 ( Suppl 2 ), S2 – S11.

Nelson, L. J. , Hart, C. H. , Wu, B. , Yang, C. , Roper, S. O. , & Jin, S. (2006). Relations between Chinese mothers' parenting practices and social withdrawal in early childhood*International Journal of Behavioral Development*, 30(3), 261 – 271.

Neumark-Sztainer, D. , Wall, M. , Perry, C. , & Story, M.

( 2003 ). Correlates of fruit and vegetable intake among adolescents: Findings from Project EAT. *Preventive Medicine*, 37 (3), 198 – 208.

Neumark-Sztainer, D. , Wall, M. , Story, M. , & van den Berg, P. ( 2008 ). Accurate parental classification of overweight adolescents' weight status: Does it matter? *Pediatrics*, 121 (6), e1495 – 1502.

Nguyen, V. T. , Larson, D. E. , Johnson, R. K. , & Goran, M. I. ( 1996 ). Fat intake and adiposity in children of lean and obese parents. *American Journal of Clinical Nutrition*, 63 (4), 507 – 513.

Nicklas, T. A. , Hayes, D. , & American Dietetic Association ( 2008 ). Position of the American dietetic association: Nutrition guidance for healthy children ages 2 to 11 Years. *Journal of the American Dietetic Association*, 108 (6), 1038 – 1047.

O'Loughlin, J. , Paradis, G. , Kishchuk, N. , Barnett, T. , & Renaud, L. ( 1999 ). Prevalence and correlates of physical activity behaviors among elementary schoolchildren in multiethnic, low income, inner-city neighborhoods in Montreal, Canada. *Annals of Epidemiology*, 9 (7), 397 – 407.

O'Rahilly, S. , & Farooqi, I. S. ( 2008 ). Human obesity: a heritable neurobehavioral disorder that is highly sensitive to environmental conditions. *Diabetes*, 57 (11), 2905 – 2910.

O' Connor, T. M. , Hughes, S. O. , Watson, K. B. , Baranowski, T. , Nicklas, T. A. , Fisher, J. O. , et al. (2010). Parenting practices are associated with fruit and vegetable consumption in pre-school children. *Public Health Nutrition* 13 (1), 91 – 101.

Ogden, C. L. , Flegal, K. M. , Carroll, M. D. , & Johnson, C. L. (2002). Prevalence and trends in overweight among US children and adolescents, 1999 – 2000. *The Journal of the American Medical Association*, 288 (14), 1728 – 1732.

Oliveria, S. A. , Ellison, R. C. , Moore, L. L. , Gillman, M. W. , Garrahie, E. J. , & Singer, M. R. (1992 ). Parent-child relationships in nutrient intake: the Framingham Children's Study. *American Journal of Clinical Nutrition*, 56 (3), 593 – 598.

Papas, M. A. , Alberg, A. J. , Ewing, R. , Helzlsouer, K. J. , Gary, T. L. , & Klassen, A. C. (2007). The built environment and obesity. *Epidemiologic Reviews*, 29 (1), 129 – 143.

Parkinson, K. N. , Tovée, M. J. , & Cohen-Tovée, E. M. (1998). Body shape perceptions of preadolescent and young adolescent children. *European Eating Disorders Review*, 6 (2), 126 – 135.

Parmenter, K. , Waller, J. , & Wardle, J. (2000). Demographic variation in nutrition knowledge in England. *Health Education Research*, 15 (2), 163 – 174.

Parsons, T. J. , Power, C. , & Manor, O. (2003). Infant feeding and obesity through the lifecourse. *Archives of Disease in Childhood*, 88 (9), 793 – 794.

Pate, R. R. , Davis, M. G. , Robinson, T. N. , Stone, E. J. , McKenzie, T. L. , & Young, J. C. (2006 ). Promoting physical activity in children and youth: a leadership role for schools: a scientific statement from the American Heart Association Council on Nutrition, Physical Activity, and Metabolism (Physical Activity Committee) in collaboration with the Councils on Cardiovascular Disease in the Young and Cardiovascular Nursing. *Circulation*, 114 (11), 1214 – 1224.

Perusse, L. , Tremblay, A. , Leblanc, C. , Cloninger, C. R. , Reich, T. , Rice, J. , et al. (1988). Familial resemblance in energy intake: contribution of genetic and environmental factors. *American Journal of Clinical Nutrition*, 47 (4), 629 – 635.

Pong, S. – l. , Johnston, J. , & Chen, V. (2009). Authoritarian Parenting and Asian Adolescent School Performance: Insights from the US and Taiwan. *International Journal of Behavioral Development*, 34 (1), 62 – 72.

Popkin, B. M. (2010). Recent dynamics suggest selected countries catching up to US obesity. *The American Journal Clinical Nutrition*, 91 (1), 284S – 288S.

Porter, C. L. , Hart, C. H. , Yang, C. , Robinson, C. C. , Olsen, S. F. , Zeng, Q. , et al. (2005). A comparative study of child temperament and parenting in Beijing, China and the western United States. *International Journal of Behavioral Development*, 29 (6), 541 – 551.

Prochaska, J. J. , Rodgers, M. W. , & James, F. S. (2002). Association of parent and peer support with adolescent physical activity. *Research Quarterly for Exercise and Sport* 73 (2), 206 – 210.

Ravussin, E. , & Bogardus, C. (1989). Relationship of genetics, age, and physical fitness to daily energy expenditure and fuel utilization. *American Journal of Clinical Nutrition*, 49 (5), 968S –975.

Reed, D. R. , Bachmanov, A. A. , Beauchamp, G. K. , Tordoff, M. G. , & Price, R. A. (1997). Heritable variation in food preferences and their contribution to obesity. *Behavior Genetics*, 27 (4), 373 –387.

Rennie, K. L. , Livingstone, M. B. E. , Wells, J. C. K. , McGloin, A. , Coward, W. A. , Prentice, A. M. , et al. (2005). Association of physical activity with body-composition indexes in children aged 6 – 8 y at varied risk of obesity. *American Journal of Clinical Nutrition*, 82 (1), 13 –20.

Rhee, K. (2008). Childhood overweight and the relationship between parent behaviors, parenting style, and family functioning. *The ANNALS of the American Academy of Political and Social Science*, 615 (1), 11 –37.

Rhee, K. , De Lago, C. W. , Arscott-Mills, T. , Mehta, S. D. , & Davis, R. K. (2005). Factors associated with parental readiness to make changes for overweight children. *Pediatrics*, 116 (1), e94 –101.

Rhee, K. , Lumeng, J. C. , Appugliese, D. P. , Kaciroti, N. , & Bradley, R. H. (2006). Parenting styles and overweight status in first grade. *Pediatrics*, 117, 2047 –2054.

Rimal, R. N. (2001). Longitudinal influences of knowledge and self-efficacy on exercise behavior: tests of a mutual reinforcement model. *Journal of Health Psychology*, 6 (1), 31 –46.

Roberts, S. B. , Savage, J. , Coward, W. A. , Chew, B. , &

Lucas, A. (1988). Energy expenditure and intake in infants born to lean and overweight mothers. *The New England Journal of Medicine*, 318 (8), 461 –466.

Robertson, W. , Friede, T. , Blissett, J. , Rudolf, M. C. J. , Wallis, M. , & Stewart-Brown, S. (2008). Pilot of "Families for Health": community-based family intervention for obesity. *Archives of Disease in Childhood*, 93 (11), 921 –928.

Robinson, T. N. (1999). Behavioural treatment of childhood and adolescent obesity. *International Journal of Obesity*, 23 (Suppl 2), S52 –57.

Saelens, B. E. , Ernst, M. M. , & Epstein, L. H. (2000). Maternal child feeding practices and obesity: A discordant sibling analysis. *International Journal of Eating Disorders*, 27 (4), 459 –463.

Saelens, B. E. , Sallis, J. F. , Black, J. B. , & Chen, D. (2003). Neighborhood-based differences in physical activity: An environment scale evaluation. *American Journal of Public Health*, 93 (9), 1552 –1558.

Sallis, J. F. , McKenzie, T. L. , Elder, J. P. , Broyles, S. L. , & Nader, P. R. (1997). Factors parents use in selecting play spaces for young children. *Archives of Pediatrics & Adolescent Medicine*, 151 (4), 414 –417.

Sallis, J. F. , Prochaska, J. J. , & Taylor, W. C. (2000). A review of correlates of physical activity of children and adolescents. *Medicine and Science in Sports and Exercise*, 32, 963.

Sallis, J. F. , Simons-Morton, B. G. , Stone, E. J. , Corbin, C. B. , Epstein, L. H. , Faucette, N. , et al. (1992). Determinants of physical activity and interventions in youth. *Medicine and Science in Sports and Exercise*, 24 (6 Suppl), S248 – S257.

Sallis, J. F. , Taylor, W. C. , Dowda, M. , Freedson, P. S. , & Pate, R. R. (2002). Correlates of vigorous physical activity for children in grades 1 through 12: comparing parent-reported and objectively measured physical activity. *Pediatric Exercise Science*, 14 (1), 30 – 44.

Salvy, S. – J. , Bowker, J. W. , Roemmich, J. N. , Romero, N. , Kieffer, E. , Paluch, R. , et al. (2008). Peer influence on children's physical activity: An experience sampling study. *Journal of Pediatric Psychology* 33 (1), 39 – 49.

Salvy, S. – J. , Howard, M. , Read, M. , & Mele, E. (2009). The presence of friends increases food intake in youth. *American Journal of Clinical Nutrition*, 90 (2), 282 – 287.

Satter, E. (2004). Children, the feeding relationship, and weight. *Maryland Medicine*, 5 (3), 26 – 28.

Savage, J. S. , Fisher, J. O. , & Birch, L. L. (2007). Parental Influence on Eating Behavior: Conception to Adolescence. *The Journal of Law, Medicine & Ethics*, 35 (1), 22 – 34.

Schaefer-Graf, U. M. , Pawliczak, J. , Passow, D. , Hartmann, R. , Rossi, R. , Buhrer, C. , et al. (2005). Birth weight and parental BMI predict overweight in children from mothers with gestational diabetes. *Diabetes Care*, 28 (7), 1745 – 1750.

Segal, K. R. , Presta, E. , & Gutin, B. (1984). Thermic effect of food during graded exercise in normal weight and obese men. *American Journal of Clinical Nutrition*, 40 (5), 995 – 1000.

Shantou municipal bureau of statistics (2010). *Statistical communique of Shantou on the* 2009 *national economic and social development*. Shantou, China: Shantou municipal bureau of statistics.

Sheu, Y. Y. (2003). *Relationship between body weight and dietary behavior of elementary school children in Taipei city and their parent's nutrition knowledge, dietary behavior, and food-related parenting style*. Taipei Medical University, Taipei.

Shi, Z. , Liena, N. , Nirmal Kumara, B. , & Holmboe-Ottesen, G. (2007). Perceptions of weight and associated factors of adolescents in Jiangsu Province, China. *Public Health Nutrition* 10, 298 – 305

Sim, J. , & Wright, C. (2000). *Research in Health Care: Concepts, Designs and Methods* Cheltenham: Stanley Thornes Ltd.

Sjoberg, R. L. , Nilsson, K. W. , & Leppert, J. (2005). Obesity, shame, and depression in school-aged children: a population-based study. *Pediatrics*, 116 (3), e389 – 392.

Skille, E. A. (2005). Individuality or cultural reproduction? adolescents' sport participation in Norway: alternative versus conventional sports. *International Review for the Sociology of Sport*, 40 (3), 307 – 320.

Skinner, A. C. , Weinberger, M. , Mulvaney, S. , Schlundt, D. , & Rothman, R. L. (2008). Accuracy of perceptions of overweight and relation to self-care behaviors among adolescents with type 2 diabetes and their parents. *Diabetes Care*, 31 (2), 227 – 229.

Smith, G. D. , Steer, C. , Leary, S. , & Ness, A. (2007). Is there an intrauterine influence on obesity? Evidence from parent child associations in the Avon Longitudinal Study of Parents and Children (ALSPAC). *Archives of Disease in Childhood*, 92 (10), 876 – 880.

Sobal, J. , & Stunkard, A. J. (1989). Socioeconomic status and obesity: a review of the literature. *Psychological Bulletin* 105 (2), 260 – 275.

Spruijt-Metz, D. , Lindquist, C. H. , Birch, L. L. , Fisher, J. O. , & Goran, M. I. (2002). Relation between mothers' child-feeding practices and children's adiposity. *American Journal of Clinical Nutrition*, 75 (3), 581 – 586.

Stattin, H. , & Kerr, M. (2000). Parental monitoring: a reinterpretation. *Child Development*, 71 (4), 1072 – 1085.

Steinberg, L. , Dornbusch, S. M. , & Brown, B. B. (1992). Ethnic differences in adolescent achievement. An ecological perspective. *The American Psychologist*, 47 (6), 723 – 729.

Stewart, L. , Chapple, J. , Hughes, A. R. , Poustie, V. , & Reilly, J. J. (2008). Parents' journey through treatment for their child's obesity: a qualitative study. *Archives of Disease in Childhood* 93 (1), 35 – 39.

Storch, E. A. , Milsom, V. A. , DeBraganza, N. , Lewin, A. B. , Geffken, G. R. , & Silverstein, J. H. (2007). Peer victimization, psychosocial adjustment, and physical activity in overweight and at-risk-for-overweight youth. *Journal of Pediatric Psychology* 32 (1), 80 – 89.

Strauss, R. S. (1997). Effects of the intrauterine environment on childhood growth. *British Medical Bulletin*, 53 (1), 81 – 95.

Strauss, R. S. , & Knight, J. (1999). Influence of the home environment on the development of obesity in children. *Pediatrics*, 103 (6), e85.

Stunkard, A. J. , Sorensen, T. I. , Hanis, C. , Teasdale, T. W. , Chakraborty, R. , Schull, W. J. , et al. (1986). An adoption study of human obesity. *The New England Journal of Medicine*, 314 (4), 193 – 198.

Sun, C. , Zhang, R. X. , Niu, J. , & Ma, J. Z. (2008). The rationale and strategies of promoting physical activity for children's health. *Journal of Nanjing Institute of Physical Education (Natural Science)*, 7 (2), 86 – 88.

Sun, Y. H. , Be, P. , & Ni, J. F. (1994). An epidemiological study on the middle school students' sports participation in Hefei. *Chinese Journal of School Health*, 15 (2), 133 – 134.

Suzanne Goodell, L. , Pierce, M. B. , Bravo, C. M. , & Ferris, A. M. (2008). Parental perceptions of overweight during early childhood. *Qualitative Health Research*, 18 (11), 1548 – 1555.

The National Institute of Child Health Human Development Study of Early Child Care and Youth Development Network (2003).

Frequency and intensity of activity of third-grade children in physical education. *Archives of Pediatrics & Adolescent Medicine*, 157 (2), 185 – 190.

Tibbs, T. , Haire-Joshu, D. , Schechtman, K. B. , Brownson, R. C. , Nanney, M. S. , Houston, C. , et al. (2001). The relationship between parental modeling, eating patterns, and dietary intake among African-American parents. *Journal of the American Dietetic Association*, 101 (5), 535 – 541.

Tordoff, M. G. (2002). Obesity by choice: the powerful influence of nutrient availability on nutrient intake. *American Journal of Physiology Regulatory Integrative Comparative Physiology*, 282 (5), R1536 – 1539.

Toschke, A. M. , Martin, R. M. , von, K. R. , Wells, J. , Smith, G. D. , & Ness, A. R. (2007). Infant feeding method and obesity: body mass index and dual-energy X-ray absorptiometry measurements at 9 – 10 y of age from the Avon Longitudinal Study of Parents and Children (ALSPAC). *American Journal of Clinical Nutrition*, 85, 1578 – 1585.

Toschke, A. M. , Montgomery, S. M. , Pfeiffer, U. , & von Kries, R. (2003). Early intrauterine exposure to tobacco-inhaled products and obesity. *American Journal Epidemiology*, 158, 1068 – 1074.

Toschke, A. M. , von Kries, R. , Beyerlein, A , & Ruckinger, S. (2008). Risk factors for childhood obesity: shift of the entire BMI distribution vs. shift of the upper tail only in a cross sectional study. *BMC Public Health*, 8 (1), 115.

Tremblay, L. , & Frigon, J. (2005). The interaction role of obesity and pubertal timing on the psychosocial adjustment of adolescent girls: Longitudinal data. *International Journal of Obesity*, 29 (10), 1204 – 1211.

Treuth, M. S. , Butte, N. F. , & Sorkin, J. D. (2003). Predictors of body fat gain in nonobese girls with a familial predisposition to obesity. *American Journal of Clinical Nutrition*, 78 (6), 1212 – 1218.

Treuth, M. S. , Butte, N. F. , & Wong, W. W. (2000). Effects of familial predisposition to obesity on energy expenditure in multiethnic prepubertal girls. *American Journal of Clinical Nutrition*, 71 (4), 893 – 900.

Trost, S. G. , Pate, R. R. , Saunders, R. , Ward, D. S. , Dowda, M. , & Felton, G. (1997). A prospective study of the determinants of physical activity in rural fifth-grade children. *Preventive Medicine*, 26 (2), 257 – 263.

Trost, S. G. , Pate, R. R. , Ward, D. S. , Saunders, R. , & Riner, W. (1999). Determinants of physical activity in active and low-active, sixth grade african-american youth. *Journal of School Health*, 69 (1), 29 – 34.

Trost, S. G. , Sallis, J. F. , Pate, R. R. , Freedson, P. S. , Taylor, W. C. , & Dowda, M. (2003). Evaluating a model of parental influence on youth physical activity. *American Journal of Preventive Medicine*, 25 (4), 277 – 282.

Tsiros, M. , Sinn, N. , Coates, A. , Howe, P. , & Buckley, J.

(2008). Treatment of adolescent overweight and obesity. *European Journal of Pediatrics*, 167 (1), 9 – 16.

van der Horst, K. , Kremers, S. , Ferreira, I. , Singh, A. , Oenema, A. , & Brug, J. (2007). Perceived parenting style and practices and the consumption of sugar-sweetened beverages by adolescents. *Health Education Research*, 22 (2), 295 – 304.

van der Horst, K. , Paw, M. J. , Twisk, J. W. , & Van Mechelen, W. (2007). A brief review on correlates of physical activity and sedentariness in youth. *Medicine and Science in Sports and Exercise*, 39 (8), 1241 – 1250.

Variyam, J. N. , & Blaylock, J. (1998). Unlocking the mystery between nutrition knowledge and diet quality. *Food Review*, 21, 21 – 28.

Variyam, J. N. , Blaylock, J. , Lin, B. – H. , Ralston, K. , & Smallwood, D. (1999). Mother's nutrition knowledge and children's dietary intakes. *American Journal of Agricultural Economics*, 81 (2), 373 – 384.

Von Kries, R. , Koletzko, B. , Sauerwald, T. , von Mutius, E. , Barnert, D. , Grunert, V. , et al. (1999). Breast feeding and obesity: cross sectional study. *British Medical Journal*, 319 (7203), 147 – 150.

Von Kries, R. , Toschke, A. M. , Koletzko, B. , & Slikker, W. , Jr. (2002). Maternal smoking during pregnancy and childhood obesity. *American Journal of Epidemiology*, 156 (10), 954 – 961.

Wada, K. , Tamakoshi, K. , Tsunekawa, T. , Otsuka, R. , Zhang, H. , Murata, C. , et al. ( 2005 ). Validity of self-reported height and weight in a Japanese workplace population. *International Journal of Obesity*, 29 (9), 1093 – 1099.

Wake, M. , Nicholson, J. M. , Hardy, P. , & Smith, K. ( 2007 ). Preschooler obesity and parenting styles of mothers and fathers: Australian national population study. *Pediatrics*, 120 (6), e1520 – 1527.

Wang, J. G. , Cui, M. C. , Su, A. F. , & Wang, F. Z. ( 2007 ). Survey on the health-related knowledge status of the parents of obesity children. *Modern Preventive Medicine*, 34, 3121 – 3122.

Wang, Y. ( 2001 ). Cross-national comparison of childhood obesity: the epidemic and the relationship between obesity and socioeconomic status. *International Journal of Epidemiology*, 30 (5), 1129 – 1136.

Wang, Y. , Monteiro, C. , & Popkin, B. M. ( 2002 ). Trends of obesity and underweight in older children and adolescents in the United States, Brazil, China, and Russia. *The American Journal of Clinical Nutrition*, 75 (6), 971 – 977.

Wang, Y. , & Zhang, Q. ( 2006 ). Are American children and adolescents of low socioeconomic status at increased risk of obesity? Changes in the association between overweight and family income between 1971 and 2002. *American Journal of Clinical Nutrition*, 84 (4), 707 – 716.

Ward, C. L. ( 2008 ). Parental Perceptions of Childhood Overweight in the Mexican American Population: An Integrative Review. *The Journal of School Nursing*, 24 (6), 407 – 416.

Wardle, J., Carnell, S., Haworth, C. M. A., & Plomin, R. (2008). Evidence for a strong genetic influence on childhood adiposity despite the force of the obesogenic environment. *American Journal of Clinical Nutrition*, 87 (2), 398 – 404.

Wardle, J., Parmenter, K., & Waller, J. (2000). Nutrition knowledge and food intake. *Appetite*, 34 (3), 269 – 275.

Warschburger, P., & Kroller, K. (2009). Maternal perception of weight status and health risks associated with obesity in children. *Pediatrics*, 124 (1), e60 – 68.

Westenhoefer, J. (2002). Establishing dietary habits during childhood for long-term weight control. *Annals of Nutrition and Metabolism*, 46 (suppl 1), 18 – 23

Whitaker, R. C., & Orzol, S. M. (2006). Obesity among us urban preschool children: relationships to race, ethnicity, and socioeconomic status. *Archives of Pediatrics & Adolescents Medicine*, 160 (6), 578 – 584.

Whitaker, R. C., Wright, J. A., Pepe, M. S., Seidel, K. D., & Dietz, W. H. (1997). Predicting obesity in young adulthood from childhood and parental obesity. *The New England Journal of Medicine*, 337 (13), 869 – 873.

Wilson, D. K., & Ampey-Thornhill, G. (2001). The role of gender and family support on dietary compliance in an African American adolescent hypertension prevention study. *Annals of Behavioral Medicine*, 23 (1), 59 – 67.

Winickoff, J. P. , Tanski, S. E. , McMillen, R. C. , Hipple, B. J. , Friebely, J. , & Healey, E. A. (2006). A national survey of the acceptability of quitlines to help parents quit smoking. *Pediatrics*, 117 (4), e695 – 700.

Woolger, C. , & Power, T. G. (1993). Parent and sport social-ization: views from the achievement literature. *Journal of Sport Behavior*, 16 (3), 171 – 189.

Worsley, A. (2002). Nutrition knowledge and food consumption: can nutrition knowledge change food behaviour? *Asia Pacific Journal of Clinical Nutrition*, 11 (suppl 3), S579 – S585.

Wright, M. S. , Wilson, D. K. , Griffin, S. , & Evans, A. (2008). A qualitative study of parental modeling and social support for physical activity in underserved adolescents. *Health Education Research*, cyn043.

Wrotniak, B. H. , Epstein, L. H. , Paluch, R. A. , & Roemmich, J. N. (2004). Parent weight change as a predictor of child weight change in family-based behavioral obesity treatment. *Archives of Pediatrics & Adolescents Medicine*, 158 (4), 342 – 347.

Wu, P. , Robinson, C. C. , Yang, C. , Hart, C. H. , Olsen, S. F. , Porter, C. L. , et al. (2002). Similarities and differences in mothers' parenting of preschoolers in China and the United States. *International Journal of Behavioral Development*, 26 (6), 481 – 491.

Wu, X. , Luke, A. , Cooper, R. S. , Zhu, X. , Kan, D. , Tayo, B. O. , et al. (2004). A genome scan among nigerians linking resting energy expenditure to chromosome 16. *Obesity*, 12 (4), 577 –581.

Xiang, P. , Lee, A. M. , & Solmon, M. A. (1997). Achievement Goals and their Correlates among American and Chinese Students in Physical Education: A Cross-Cultural Analysis. *Journal of Cross-Cultural Psychology*, 28 (6), 645 –660.

Xiao, T. F. , Yang, Y. F. , & He, H. L. (2001). Case control study on family factors in children with simple obesity. *China Public Health*, 17 (11), 1002 –1003.

Xie, B. , Chou, C. –P. , Spruijt-Metz, D. , Reynolds, K. , Clark, F. , Palmer, P. H. , et al. (2006). Weight perception and weight-related sociocultural and behavioral factors in Chinese adolescents. *Preventive Medicine*, 42 (3), 229.

Xie, B. , Liu, C. , Chou, C. – P. , Xia, J. , Spruijt-Metz, D. , Gong, J. , et al. (2003). Weight perception and psychological factors in Chinese adolescents. *The Journal of Adolescent Health*, 33 (3), 202 –210.

Xu, Y. , Farver, J. A. M. , Zhang, Z. , Zeng, Q. , Yu, L. , & Cai, B. (2005). Mainland Chinese parenting styles and parent-child interaction. *International Journal of Behavioral Development*, 29 (6), 524 –531.

Yang, X. L. , Telama, R. , & Laakso, L. (1996). Parents' physical activity, socioeconomic status and education as predictors of physical activity and sport among children and youths – A 12 – year follow – up study. *International Review for the Sociology of Sport*, 31 (3), 273 –291.

Yau, J. , & Smetana, J. G. (1996). Adolescent-parent conflict among Chinese adolescents in Hong Kong *Child Development*, 67 (3), 1262 – 1275.

Yeung, D. C. S. , & Hui, S. C. (2007). Evaluation of the 1993 reference criteria for assessing the prevalence of childhood obesity in Hong Kong. *Medicine and Science in Sports and Exercise*, 39 (5, suppl. ), S378.

Young, K. M. , Northern, J. J. , Lister, K. M. , Drummond, J. A. , & O'Brien, W. H. (2007). A meta-analysis of family-behavioral weight-loss treatments for children. *Clinical Psychology Review*, 27 (2), 240 –249.

Yu, S. W. K. , & Chau, R. C. M. (1997). The sexual division of care in mainland China and Hong Kong. *International Journal of Urban and Regional Research*, 21 (4), 607 –619.

Yu, Y. , Li, H. , Xia, X. L. , Tong, F. , & Sun, S. Y. (2002). Influence of parental overweight on the development of childhood obesity. *China Public Health* 18, 1463 – 1464.

Zask, A. , van Beurden, E. , Barnett, L. , Brooks, L. O. , & Dietrich, U. C. (2001). Active school playgrounds—myth or reality? Results of the "Move It Groove It" project. *Preventive Medicine*, 33 (5), 402 –408.

Zhou, B. F. , & Cooperative Meta-Analysis Group of the Working Group on Obesity in China (2002). Predictive values of body mass index and waist circumference for risk factors of certain related diseases in Chinese adults—study on optimal cut-off points of body mass index and waist circumference in Chinese adults. *Biomedical and Environmental Sciences*, 15 (1), 83 – 96.

# 附　件

## 附件　I

### 研究同意书

亲爱的家长：

　　您好！

　　香港中文大学一个科研小组正在进行调查，期望了解您孩子的一些健康信息。这项研究计划由许世全教授指导，由本人执行。

　　本次研究拟邀请广东省汕头市和江西省赣州市各1000名初一和初二的学生及其父亲或母亲参与。在调查过程中，将邀请同学和家长各填写一份问卷，并测量学生的身高体重。学生问卷填写和身高体重测量将安排与下午第三节自习课进行，整个过程需要大概30－45分钟，不会影响学生的正常教学。家长问卷由学生带回家中，请家长填写后再由学生带回学校，填写该问卷需要大约 10 – 20 分钟。完成调查后，学生将得到本次调查的纪念品一份。

参与本次研究纯属自愿性质，学生和家长可自行决定是否参与，也可在调查过程中自由退出。本次研究所收集的个人资料仅作为整体统计计算，个人信息不会公开，个人的测试结果也将绝对保密。

烦请您填妥回条，并嘱咐子女与翌日交还负责老师。研究人员与负责老师将会直接与接受调查的学生联络，并解释和安排研究。如得到您的同意，不胜感激！

如有任何疑问，请向本次研究协调员温煦先生查询！

香港中文大学　　温煦 博士研究生

电话：（86）15907976103（大陆）

（852）67605816（香港）

电邮：wenxu@cuhk.edu.hk

## 同意书回条

研究协调员　温煦先生：

本人＿＿＿＿＿＿＿（家长姓名）及子女＿＿＿＿＿＿＿
（子女姓名）

□ 同意（联络电话：＿＿＿＿＿＿＿）

□ 不同意

一起参加该项研究。本人已详阅此同意书，并清楚研究的
目的和内容。

家长签名：＿＿＿＿＿＿＿　　　　日期＿＿＿＿＿＿＿

子女签名：＿＿＿＿＿＿＿　　　　日期＿＿＿＿＿＿＿

# 附件 II

学生问卷（男生）　　　　　　编号：＿＿＿＿＿＿

\*\*\*\*\*\*\*\*\*\*\*\*\*\*\*\*\*\*\*\*\*\*\*\*\*\*\*\*\*\*\*\*\*\*\*\*\*\*\*\*\*\*\*\*

身高：＿＿＿＿＿＿厘米　　　　体重：＿＿＿＿＿＿公斤

（此部分请由工作人员填写）

\*\*\*\*\*\*\*\*\*\*\*\*\*\*\*\*\*\*\*\*\*\*\*\*\*\*\*\*\*\*\*\*\*\*\*\*\*\*\*\*\*\*\*\*

亲爱的同学：

你好！这份问卷的目的是想了解一些你的健康信息。**请注意这不是考试，答案没有对错之分。**同时问卷是不记名的，你所填写的个人资料也会**绝对保密。请你仔细阅读，依照你自己的想法和实际情况来选择！**

问卷填写说明：请在情况相符前面的"□"内打"√"，或在横在线相应填写文字。无法回答或者不方便的回答的问题，可以在"不能回答"前面的"○"打"√"。如有填写错误，请在划错"√"处画"×"，再另选新答案。**除有特殊标明为多选题外，其他选择题均为单项选择题。**如对问卷有任何疑问可以随时问我们的工作人员！谢谢你的配合！并祝你学习进步！

基本数据：

性别：□ 男生　□ 女生　　出生年月：＿＿＿＿年＿＿＿＿月

**第一部分**

1. 请选择以下亲人平时是否和你住在一起？**（可多选）**。

　□母亲；□ 父亲；□ 继母；□ 继父；□ 奶奶；□ 爷爷；
□ 外婆；□ 外公

2. 请选择下面哪幅图最像你？

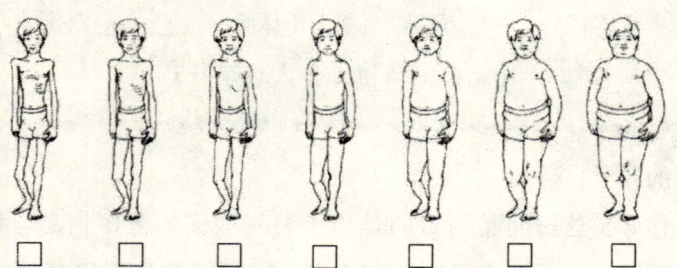

　□　　□　　□　　□　　□　　□　　□

3. 请选择下面哪幅图是你希望自己的样子？

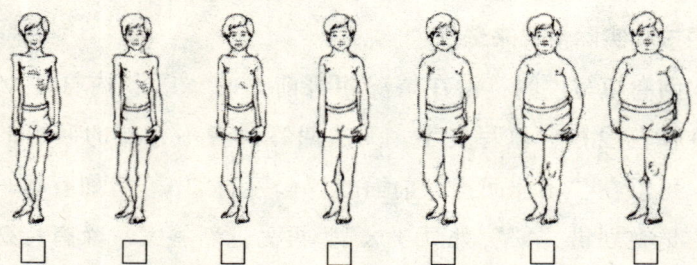

　□　　□　　□　　□　　□　　□　　□

4. 请选择下面哪幅图最像你爸爸的外形？

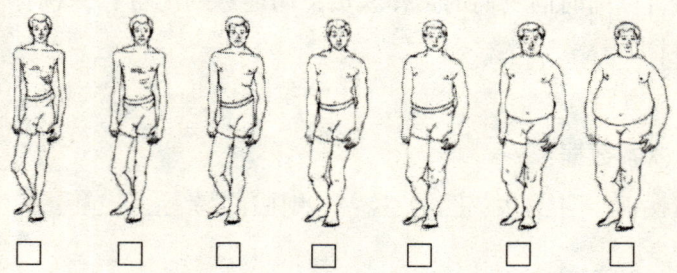

　□　　□　　□　　□　　□　　□　　□

5. 请选择下面哪幅图最像你妈妈的外形？

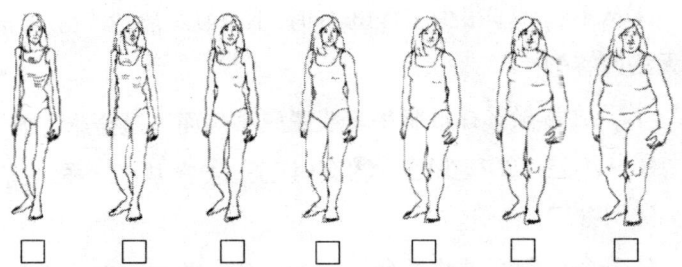

□ □ □ □ □ □ □

6. 请选择下面哪幅图是你希望自己长大后的样子？

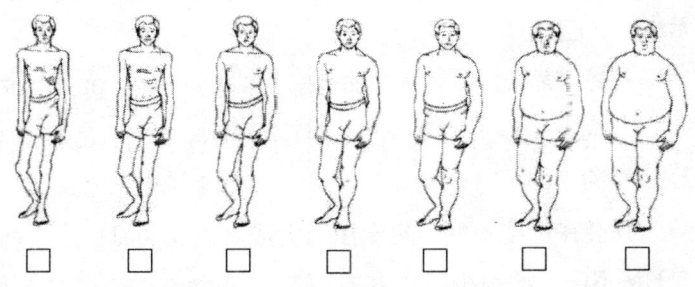

□ □ □ □ □ □ □

7. 在过去的一年中，你是否曾刻意地通过节食或运动减肥？假如有，时间有多长？

□ 1 从没有　　□ 2 不到一周　　□ 3 不到一个月 □ 4 一个月到三个月（不包括三个月）　□ 5 三个月到半年（不包括半年）□ 6 坚持了半年或半年以上

**第二部分**　请在下列叙述中挑选出一个最能反映你过去一年总体上的饮食情况。

1. 我每天至少吃三份蔬菜（煮熟蔬菜一份约为 1/2 饭碗的量）

①从不□　②很少□　③有时□　④常常□　⑤总是□⑥无法回答□

2. 我每天至少吃两份水果（一份约一个中等大的苹果或香蕉）

①从不□　②很少□　③有时□　④常常□　⑤总是□
⑥无法回答□

3. 我会尽量选择低脂牛奶或脱脂牛奶而不是全脂牛奶

①从不□　②很少□　③有时□　④常常□　⑤总是□
⑥无法回答□

4. 我每天都会油炸类食品（如油条、煎饺，椒盐排条等）

①从不□　②很少□　③有时□　④常常□　⑤总是□
⑥无法回答□

5. 我每天都喝含糖饮料（如可乐、芬达、雪碧，鲜橙多等）

①从不□　②很少□　③有时□　④常常□　⑤总是□
⑥无法回答□

6. 我会在情绪不好、感觉压力大或者无聊的时候吃东西

①从不□　②很少□　③有时□　④常常□　⑤总是□
⑥无法回答□

7. 我每周至少吃两次西式快餐（汉堡、批萨，炸鸡等）

①从不□　②很少□　③有时□　④常常□　⑤总是□
⑥无法回答□

8. 我喝汤的时候，假如汤上有一层油，会设法去掉油再喝

①从不□　②很少□　③有时□　④常常□　⑤总是□
⑥无法回答□

9. 我吃饭的时候，经常会用卤汁或菜汤拌着饭吃

①从不□　②很少□　③有时□　④常常□　⑤总是□
⑥无法回答□

10. 我吃饭口味比较清淡（很少吃油腻，咸辣的食物）

①从不□　②很少□　③有时□　④常常□　⑤总是□

⑥无法回答□

11. 我吃饭时，假如有合口味的菜，会比平时多吃一点

①从不□　②很少□　③有时□　④常常□　⑤总是□

⑥无法回答□

12. 我每天都会吃早餐

①从不□　②很少□　③有时□　④常常□　⑤总是□

⑥无法回答□


## 第三部分

请分别选择以下描述中选择最符合你父母行为的选项。

1. 我爸爸/妈妈不让我自己决定事情该怎么做，总是吩咐我该怎么做。

爸爸：①一点不像□　②有点像□　③比较像□　④非常像□　⑤不能回答□

妈妈：①一点不像□　②有点像□　③比较像□　④非常像□　⑤不能回答□

2. 我爸爸/妈妈制定规矩（如：我可以几点钟出去玩）从来不考虑我的想法

爸爸：①一点不像□　②有点像□　③比较像□　④非常像□　⑤不能回答□

妈妈：①一点不像□　②有点像□　③比较像□　④非常像□　⑤不能回答□

3. 当我心情不好时，我爸爸/妈妈总能让我感觉好起来

爸爸：①一点不像□　②有点像□　③比较像□　④非常像□　⑤不能回答□

妈妈：①一点不像□　②有点像□　③比较像□　④非常像□　⑤不能回答□

4. 我爸爸/妈妈总是太忙都没有空跟我聊聊天

爸爸：①一点不像□　②有点像□　③比较像□　④非常像□　⑤不能回答□

妈妈：①一点不像□　②有点像□　③比较像□　④非常像□　⑤不能回答□

5. 我爸爸/妈妈总会倾听我说的话

爸爸：①一点不像□　②有点像□　③比较像□　④非常像□　⑤不能回答□

妈妈：①一点不像□　②有点像□　③比较像□　④非常像□　⑤不能回答□

6. 在我爸爸/妈妈面前，我可以说真心话，表现真实的自己，不需要任何遮掩。

爸爸：①一点不像□　②有点像□　③比较像□　④非常像□　⑤不能回答□

妈妈：①一点不像□　②有点像□　③比较像□　④非常像□　⑤不能回答□

7. 当我表现好的时候，我爸爸/妈妈会表扬我

爸爸：①一点不像□　②有点像□　③比较像□　④非常像□　⑤不能回答□

妈妈：①一点不像□　②有点像□　③比较像□　④非常像□　⑤不能回答□

8. 我爸爸/妈妈愿意听我说我遇到的困难。

爸爸：①一点不像□　②有点像□　③比较像□　④非常像□　⑤不能回答□

妈妈：①一点不像□　②有点像□　③比较像□　④非常像□　⑤不能回答□

9. 我的表现无论好坏，我爸爸/妈妈都喜欢。

爸爸：①一点不像□　②有点像□　③比较像□　④非常像□　⑤不能回答□

妈妈：①一点不像□　②有点像□　③比较像□　④非常像□　⑤不能回答□

10. 我爸爸/妈妈制定的规矩（如：我可以几点钟出去玩），我必须遵守

爸爸：①一点不像□　②有点像□　③比较像□　④非常像□　⑤不能回答□

妈妈：①一点不像□　②有点像□　③比较像□　④非常像□　⑤不能回答□

11. 我爸爸/妈妈会叮嘱我必须几点几点前回家

爸爸：①一点不像□　②有点像□　③比较像□　④非常像□　⑤不能回答□

妈妈：①一点不像□　②有点像□　③比较像□　④非常像□　⑤不能回答□

12. 我去什么地方必须得告诉我爸爸/妈妈

爸爸：①一点不像□　②有点像□　③比较像□　④非常像□　⑤不能回答□

妈妈：①一点不像□　②有点像□　③比较像□　④非常像□　⑤不能回答□

**13. 我爸爸/妈妈总是让我准时睡觉**

爸爸：①一点不像□　②有点像□　③比较像□　④非常像□　⑤不能回答□

妈妈：①一点不像□　②有点像□　③比较像□　④非常像□　⑤不能回答□

**14. 我爸爸/妈妈会过问我和朋友们都干了些什么**

爸爸：①一点不像□　②有点像□　③比较像□　④非常像□　⑤不能回答□

妈妈：①一点不像□　②有点像□　③比较像□　④非常像□　⑤不能回答□

**15. 我爸爸/妈妈清楚我放学以后去什么地方**

爸爸：①一点不像□　②有点像□　③比较像□　④非常像□　⑤不能回答□

妈妈：①一点不像□　②有点像□　③比较像□　④非常像□　⑤不能回答□

**16. 我爸爸/妈妈会检查我是否做完我的家庭作业**

爸爸：①一点不像□　②有点像□　③比较像□　④非常像□　⑤不能回答□

妈妈：①一点不像□　②有点像□　③比较像□　④非常像□　⑤不能回答□

## CUHK 学生课余运动量评级问卷

请您于下列 0 - 10 的等级中，选取**其中一个等级**代表您过去一年内**平均每星期**的运动量，然后填入下面方格中：（**请参考下列附表中有关低强度、中等强度、及剧烈运动的例子**）

**低强度运动**：是简单可以应付自如的运动，呼吸心跳没有明显加速，没有出汗。

**中等强度运动**：做这类运动时，呼吸和心跳稍微加快，轻微出汗，但不觉辛苦。

**剧烈运动**：做这类运动时，呼吸和心跳很快，大量出汗，觉得很辛苦。

**从下表 0 - 10 的等级中，只选一个等级填入此方格——→** ☐

---

**没有运动习惯者，选 0 至 2**

0—完全没有任何运动，大部分时间是坐着或睡觉。

1—除了在体育课有少许活动外，其余所有时间都没有运动。

2— 除了上本育课时有积极参与运动外，其余所有时间都没有运动。

**除了上体育课有运动外，平时间中有运动习惯者，选 3 至 6**

3—每星期都有一至两次 20 分钟以上低强度运动。

4—每星期都有三次以上 20 分钟以上低强度运动。

5—差不多每天都有一次 20 分钟以上低强度运动。

6—每星期都有一至两次 20 分钟以上中等强度运动。

**除了上体育课有运动外，平时经常有运动习惯者，选 7 至 10**

7—每星期都有三次至五次中等强度运动（每次 20 分钟或以上）。

8—差不多每天都有中等强度运动（每次 20 分钟或以上）。

9—每星期都有不多三次剧烈运动（每次 20 分钟或以上）。

10—差不多每天都有剧烈运动（每次 20 分钟或以上）。

**＊附表：低强度、中等强度、及剧烈运动的例子**

| | 低强度运动 | 中等运动 | 剧烈运动 |
|---|---|---|---|
| 体育运动 | 速度很慢的散步、遛狗 | 散步（健步行，速度较快）慢跑 | 快速跑（感觉很辛苦） |
| | 保龄球 | 骑自行车 | 剧烈的篮球、足球比赛 |
| | 排球练习 | 投篮练习嬉戏型式的游泳 | 连续游泳（不间断） |
| | 节奏较慢的舞蹈（如慢舞或华尔兹） | 舞蹈或健美操（低冲击性的健美操） | 越野跑步、定向越野 |
| | 玩飞碟 | 羽毛球练习 | |
| 家居活动 | 下楼梯 | 上下楼梯（混合） | 搬运大型东西或家具上楼梯 |
| | 逛街（较轻松、速度较慢、没有携带大量物品） | 用手或跪地型式的抹地；较辛苦的家务，如抹窗或洗车 | 剧烈的运动（如：连续做俯卧撑） |
| | 做比较轻松的家务，如抹地吸尘或清洁家居 | 家中的运动，如柔软体操、仰卧起坐等 | |
| | 站立或轻量的玩耍 | 携带不超过 15 斤物品步行上楼梯 | |
| | 在家中行走及搬动轻的物品 | 在游乐场游玩（有一定体力消耗的项目） | |
| | 弹吉他或其他乐器（站立） | | |

## 男性生殖器官发育的自我评估

以下各图代表男性生殖器官发育的 5 个不同阶段（包抱阴茎、阴囊和睪丸）。

请细看以下各图及细阅图下文字，据你自己身体发育情况，选择你最接近的图前的"□"里打"√"。

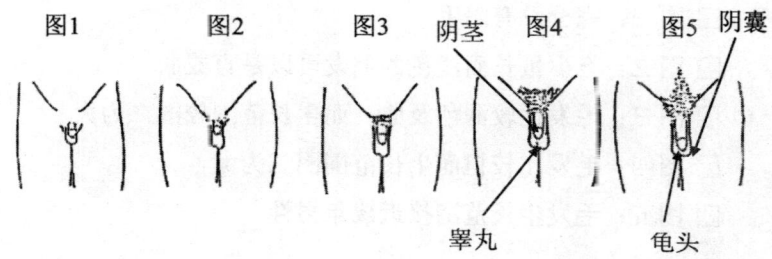

□ 图一：睪丸、阴囊及阴茎的大小和形状跟小孩子一样

□ 图二：睪丸和阴囊比较大，而阴囊较前向下松弛及阴囊表皮有改变。阴茎也比前较大。

□ 图三：阴茎长度增加，而睪丸及阴囊也比较图二多向下松弛。

□ 图四：阴茎长度继续增加及变粗，龟头也变大。阴囊比前深色，睪丸体积增大。

□ 图五：阴茎、阴囊及睪丸的大小和形状至成年男性模样。

## 男性阴毛发育的自我评估

以下各图代表男性阴毛生长的不同分布及数量。请细看以下各图及细阅图下文字，据你自己身体发育情况，选择你最接近的图前的"□"里打"√"。(在选择适当的图画时，请根据阴毛的分布及数量，而不是根据生殖器官的大小而作出决定)。

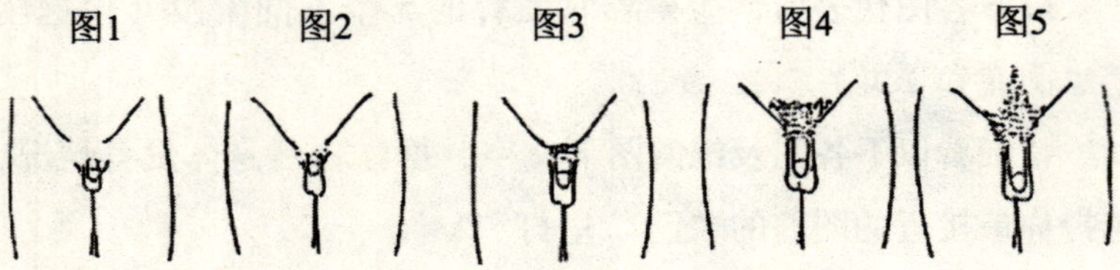

图1　　　　图2　　　　图3　　　　图4　　　　图5

□ 图一：完全没有阴毛
□ 图二：有少量长而浅色的毛发可以是直或曲
□ 图三：毛发比较深色及曲，而生长范围较图二为大
□ 图四：毛发比较粗而生长范围图三为大
□ 图五：毛发生长范围接近成年男性

# 附件 Ⅲ

学生问卷（女生）　　　　　　　编号：＿＿＿＿＿＿＿

＊＊＊＊＊＊＊＊＊＊＊＊＊＊＊＊＊＊＊＊＊＊＊＊＊＊＊＊＊＊＊＊＊＊＊＊＊＊＊＊

身高：＿＿＿＿＿＿＿厘米　　　　体重：＿＿＿＿＿＿＿公斤

（此部分请由工作人员填写）

＊＊＊＊＊＊＊＊＊＊＊＊＊＊＊＊＊＊＊＊＊＊＊＊＊＊＊＊＊＊＊＊＊＊＊＊＊＊＊＊

亲爱的同学：

你好！这份问卷的目的是想了解一些你的健康信息。**请注意这不是考试，答案没有对错之分**。同时问卷是**不记名**的，你所填写的个人资料也会**绝对保密。请你仔细阅读，依照你自己的想法和实际情况来选择**！

问卷填写说明：请在情况相符前面的"□"内打"√"，或在横在线相应填写文字。无法回答或者不方便的回答的问题，可以在"不能回答"前面的"○"打"√"。如有填写错误，请在划错"√"处画"×"，再另选新答案。**除有特殊标明为多选题外，其他选择题均为单项选择题**。如对问卷有任何疑问可以随时问我们的工作人员！谢谢你的配合！并祝你学习进步！

基本数据：

性别：□ 男生　□ 女生　　出生年月：＿＿＿＿年＿＿＿＿月

181

第一部分

1. 请选择以下亲人平时是否和你住在一起？（**可多选**）。

□ 母亲；□ 父亲；□ 继母；□ 继父；□ 奶奶；□ 爷爷；
□ 外婆；□ 外公

2. 请选择下面哪幅图最像你？

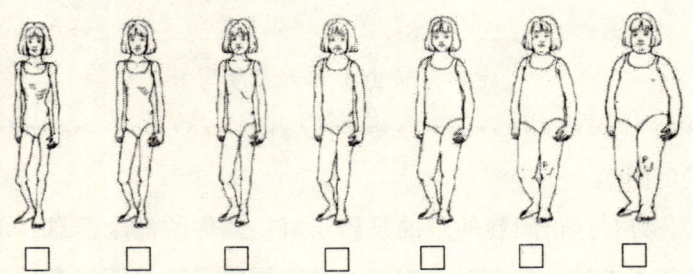

□　　□　　□　　□　　□　　□　　□

3. 请选择下面哪幅图是你希望自己的样子？

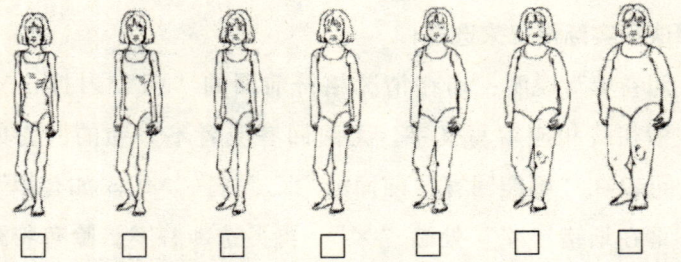

□　　□　　□　　□　　□　　□　　□

4. 请选择下面哪幅图最像你爸爸的外形？

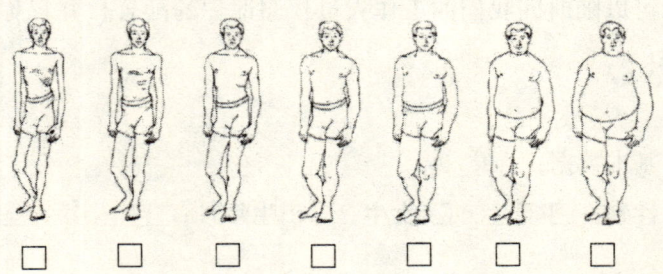

□　　□　　□　　□　　□　　□　　□

5. 请选择下面哪幅图最像你妈妈的外形？

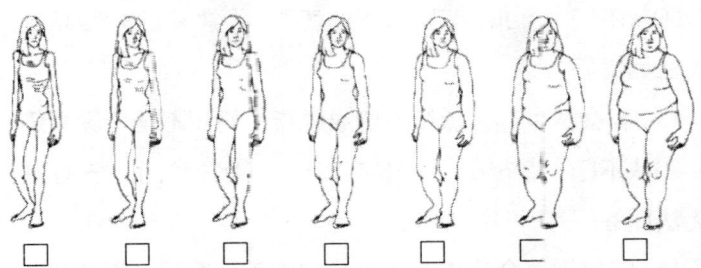

☐　☐　☐　☐　☐　☐　☐

6. 请选择下面哪幅图是你希望自己长大后的样子？

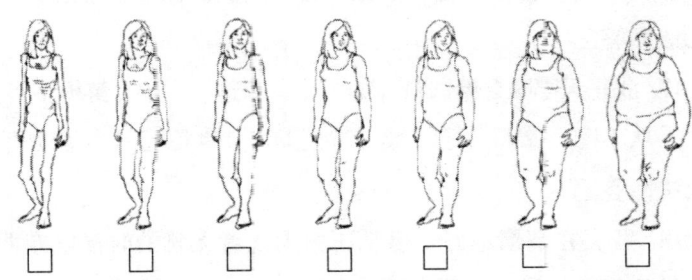

☐　☐　☐　☐　☐　☐　☐

7. 在过去的一年中，你是否曾刻意地通过节食或运动减肥？假如有，时间有多长？

☐ 1 从没有　☐ 2 不到一周　☐ 3 不到一个月　☐ 4 一个月到三个月（不包括三个月）　☐ 5 三个月到半年（不包括半年）　☐ 6 坚持了半年或半年以上

**第二部分**　请在下列叙述中挑选出一个最能反映你过去一年总体上的饮食情况。

13. 我每天至少吃三份蔬菜（煮熟蔬菜一份约为 1/2 饭碗的量）

②从不☐　②很少☐　③有时☐　④常常☐　⑤总是☐
⑥无法回答☐

**14. 我每天至少吃两份水果（一份约一个中等大的苹果或香蕉）**

①从不□　②很少□　③有时□　④常常□　⑤总是□
⑥无法回答□

**15. 我会尽量选择低脂牛奶或脱脂牛奶而不是全脂牛奶**

①从不□　②很少□　③有时□　④常常□　⑤总是□
⑥无法回答□

**16. 我每天都会油炸类食品（如油条、煎饺，椒盐排条等）**

①从不□　②很少□　③有时□　④常常□　⑤总是□
⑥无法回答□

**17. 我每天都喝含糖饮料（如可乐、芬达、雪碧，鲜橙多等）**

①从不□　②很少□　③有时□　④常常□　⑤总是□
⑥无法回答□

**18. 我会在情绪不好、感觉压力大或者无聊的时候吃东西**

①从不□　②很少□　③有时□　④常常□　⑤总是□
⑥无法回答□

**19. 我每周至少吃两次西式快餐（汉堡、批萨，炸鸡等）**

①从不□　②很少□　③有时□　④常常□　⑤总是□
⑥无法回答□

**20. 我喝汤的时候，假如汤上有一层油，会设法去掉油再喝**

①从不□　②很少□　③有时□　④常常□　⑤总是□
⑥无法回答□

**21. 我吃饭的时候，经常会用卤汁或菜汤拌着饭吃**

①从不□　②很少□　③有时□　④常常□　⑤总是□
⑥无法回答□

**22. 我吃饭口味比较清淡（很少吃油腻，咸辣的食物）**

①从不☐  ②很少☐  ③有时☐  ④常常☐  ⑤总是☐
⑥无法回答☐

**23. 我吃饭时，假如有合口味的菜，会比平时多吃一点**

①从不☐  ②很少☐  ③有时☐  ④常常☐  ⑤总是☐
⑥无法回答☐

**24. 我每天都会吃早餐**

①从不☐  ②很少☐  ③有时☐  ④常常☐  ⑤总是☐
⑥无法回答☐


**第三部分**

请分别选择以下描述中选择最符合你父母行为的选项。

**4. 我爸爸/妈妈不让我自己决定事情该怎么做，总是吩咐我
该怎么做。**

爸爸：①一点不像☐  ②有点像☐  ③比较像☐  ④非常
像☐  ⑤不能回答☐

妈妈：①一点不像☐  ②有点像☐  ③比较像☐  ④非常
像☐  ⑤不能回答☐

**5. 我爸爸/妈妈制定规矩（如：我可以几点钟出去玩）从
来不考虑我的想法**

爸爸：①一点不像☐  ②有点像☐  ③比较像☐  ④非常
像☐  ⑤不能回答☐

妈妈：①一点不像☐  ②有点像☐  ③比较像☐  ④非常
像☐  ⑤不能回答☐

6. 当我心情不好时，我爸爸/妈妈总能让我感觉好起来

爸爸：①一点不像□　②有点像□　③比较像□　④非常像□　⑤不能回答□

妈妈：①一点不像□　②有点像□　③比较像□　④非常像□　⑤不能回答□

4. 我爸爸/妈妈总是太忙都没有空跟我聊聊天

爸爸：①一点不像□　②有点像□　③比较像□　④非常像□　⑤不能回答□

妈妈：①一点不像□　②有点像□　③比较像□　④非常像□　⑤不能回答□

5. 我爸爸/妈妈总会倾听我说的话

爸爸：①一点不像□　②有点像□　③比较像□　④非常像□　⑤不能回答□

妈妈：①一点不像□　②有点像□　③比较像□　④非常像□　⑤不能回答□

6. 在我爸爸/妈妈面前，我可以说真心话，表现真实的自己，不需要任何遮掩。

爸爸：①一点不像□　②有点像□　③比较像□　④非常像□　⑤不能回答□

妈妈：①一点不像□　②有点像□　③比较像□　④非常像□　⑤不能回答□

7. 当我表现好的时候，我爸爸/妈妈会表扬我

爸爸：①一点不像□　②有点像□　③比较像□　④非常像□　⑤不能回答□

妈妈：①一点不像□　②有点像□　③比较像□　④非常像□　⑤不能回答□

8. 我爸爸/妈妈愿意听我说我遇到的困难。

爸爸：①一点不像□　②有点像□　③比较像□　④非常像□　⑤不能回答□

妈妈：①一点不像□　②有点像□　③比较像□　④非常像□　⑤不能回答□

9. 我的表现无论好坏，我爸爸/妈妈都喜欢。

爸爸：①一点不像□　②有点像□　③比较像□　④非常像□　⑤不能回答□

妈妈：①一点不像□　②有点像□　③比较像□　④非常像□　⑤不能回答□

10. 我爸爸/妈妈制定的规矩（如：我可以几点钟出去玩），我必须遵守

爸爸：①一点不像□　②有点像□　③比较像□　④非常像□　⑤不能回答□

妈妈：①一点不像□　②有点像□　③比较像□　④非常像□　⑤不能回答□

11. 我爸爸/妈妈会叮嘱我必须几点几点前回家

爸爸：①一点不像□　②有点像□　③比较像□　④非常像□　⑤不能回答□

妈妈：①一点不像□　②有点像□　③比较像□　④非常像□　⑤不能回答□

12. 我去什么地方必须得告诉我爸爸/妈妈

爸爸：①一点不像□　②有点像□　③比较像□　④非常像□　⑤不能回答□

妈妈：①一点不像□　②有点像□　③比较像□　④非常像□　⑤不能回答□

13. 我爸爸/妈妈总是让我准时睡觉

爸爸：①一点不像□　②有点像□　③比较像□　④非常像□　⑤不能回答□

妈妈：①一点不像□　②有点像□　③比较像□　④非常像□　⑤不能回答□

14. 我爸爸/妈妈会过问我和朋友们都干了些什么

爸爸：①一点不像□　②有点像□　③比较像□　④非常像□　⑤不能回答□

妈妈：①一点不像□　②有点像□　③比较像□　④非常像□　⑤不能回答□

15. 我爸爸/妈妈清楚我放学以后去什么地方

爸爸：①一点不像□　②有点像□　③比较像□　④非常像□　⑤不能回答□

妈妈：①一点不像□　②有点像□　③比较像□　④非常像□　⑤不能回答□

16. 我爸爸/妈妈会检查我是否做完我的家庭作业

爸爸：①一点不像□　②有点像□　③比较像□　④非常像□　⑤不能回答□

妈妈：①一点不像□　②有点像□　③比较像□　④非常像□　⑤不能回答□

## CUHK 学生课余运动量评级问卷

请您于下列 0 – 10 的等级中，选取**其中一个等级**代表您过去一年内**平均每星期**的运动量，然后填入下面方格中：（**请参考下列附表中有关低强度、中等强度、及剧烈运动的例子**）

**低强度运动**：是简单可以应付自如的运动，呼吸心跳没有明显加速，没有出汗。

**中等强度运动**：做这类运动时，呼吸和心跳稍微加快，轻微出汗，但不觉辛苦。

**剧烈运动**：做这类运动时，呼吸和心跳很快，大量出汗，觉得很辛苦。

**从下表 0 – 10 的等级中，只选一个等级填入此方格**──────→ ☐

---

**没有运动习惯者，选 0 至 2**

　　0—完全没有任何运动，大部分时间是坐着或睡觉。

　　1—除了在体育课有少许活动外，其余所有时间都没有运动。

　　2—除了上体育课时有积极参与运动外，其余所有时间都没有运动。

**除了上体育课有运动外，平时间中有运动习惯者，选 3 至 6**

　　3—每星期都有一至两次 20 分钟以上低强度运动。

　　4—每星期都有三次以上 20 分钟以上低强度运动。

　　5—差不多每天都有一次 20 分钟以上低强度运动。

　　6—每星期都有一至两次 20 分钟以上中等强度运动。

**除了上体育课有运动外，平时经常有运动习惯者，选 7 至 10**

　　7—每星期都有三次至五次中等强度运动（每次 20 分钟或以上）。

　　8—差不多每天都有中等强度运动（每次 20 分钟或以上）。

　　9—每星期都有不多于三次剧烈运动（每次 20 分钟或以上）。

　　10—差不多每天都有剧烈运动（每次 20 分钟或以上）。

**＊附表：低强度、中等强度、及剧烈运动的例子**

| | 低强度运动 | 中等运动 | 剧烈运动 |
|---|---|---|---|
| 体育运动 | 速度很慢的散步、遛狗 | 散步（健步行，速度较快）<br>慢跑 | 快速跑（感觉很辛苦） |
| | 保龄球 | 骑自行车 | 剧烈的篮球、足球比赛 |
| | 排球练习 | 投篮练习<br>嬉戏型式的游泳 | 连续游泳（不间断） |
| | 节奏较慢的舞蹈（如慢舞或华尔兹） | 舞蹈或健美操（低冲击性的健美操） | 越野跑步、定向越野 |
| | 玩飞碟 | 羽毛球练习 | |
| 家居活动 | 下楼梯 | 上下楼梯（混合） | 搬运大型东西或家具上楼梯 |
| | 逛街（较轻松、速度较慢、没有携带大量物品） | 用手或跪地型式的抹地；较辛苦的家务，如抹窗或洗车 | 剧烈的运动（如：连续做俯卧撑） |
| | 做比较轻松的家务，如抹地吸尘或清洁家居 | 家中的运动，如柔软体操、仰卧起坐等 | |
| | 站立或轻量的玩耍 | 携带不超过 15 斤物品步行上楼梯 | |
| | 在家中行走及搬动轻的物品 | 在游乐场游玩（有一定体力消耗的项目） | |
| | 弹吉他或其他乐器（站立） | | |

## 女性乳房发育的自我评估

　　以下各图代表女性乳房发育的 5 个不同阶段。请细看以各图及细阅图下文字，根据你自己乳房发育的情况，选择你最接近的图前的"□"里打"√"。

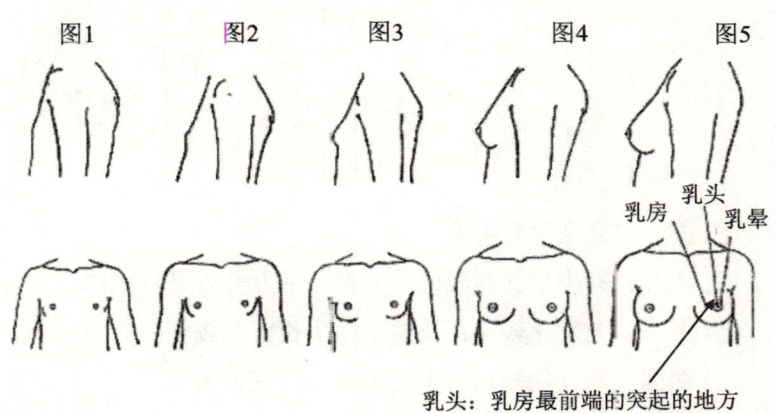

乳头：乳房最前端的突起的地方
乳晕：乳头外围粉红色略突起的部分

　　□ 图一：乳头有些微突起，乳房其他部份则平坦。

　　□ 图二：乳头比图一较突起，乳晕比图一为大，乳房有些微涨起。

　　□ 图三：乳晕和乳房比图二更大，但乳晕没有突起现象。

　　□ 图四：乳晕及乳头从乳房的轮廓中突起。（请注意，有些女性没有图四的现象，而由图三直接发展至图五）。

　　□ 图五：乳房完全发育至成年女性样，乳头呈现突出，但乳晕变为平坦。

## 女性阴毛发育的自我评估

　　以下各图代表女性阴毛生长的不同分布及数量。请细看以下各图及细阅图下文字，根据你自己身体发育情况，选择你最接近的图前的"□"里打"√"。

图1　　　　图2　　　　图3　　　　图4　　　　图5

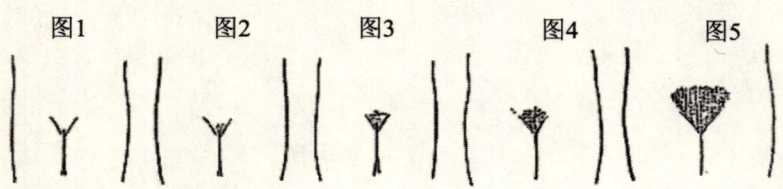

□ 图一：完全没有阴毛

□ 图二：有少量长而浅色的毛发，毛发可以是直或曲。

□ 图三：毛发比较深色及曲，而生长范围较图二为大

□ 图四：毛发比较粗而生长范围较图三为大

□ 图五：毛发生长范围接近成年女性

# 附件 Ⅳ

**此部分内容请孩子的父亲或母亲填写**　　编号_____

亲爱的家长：

您好！这份问卷是想了解一些您孩子的健康信息，以作为今后儿童青少年健康政策制订的依据。请您仔细阅读问卷内容，依据您的实际情况填写。**本问卷的问题，没有对错之分，问卷不记名，所填写的个人资料也绝对保密，请您放心。请注意，假如您有多名孩子，本问卷中"孩子"是指参加本次调查的孩子。**问卷填写完，请交由子女带回学校。承蒙您百忙中填写问卷，不胜感激！谢谢您的协助与参与！并祝愉快！

**填写说明：**请在情况相符前面的"□"内打"√"，或在"_____"上填写相应的数字。

**第一部分**

1. 您与孩子旳关系
□ 母亲　　□ 父亲　　□ 继母　　□ 继父　　□ 其他亲属或朋友

2. 您家的常住人口有_____人，有_____个孩子

3. 您孩子出生时的体重是_____公斤（或_____斤_____两），或 □ 我记不得了

4. 您孩子出生后母乳喂养（完全依靠母乳喂养，没有添加米糊、菜泥等辅食）的时间为：
_____个月或 □ 我记不得.

5. 孩子父亲现在的身高_____厘米　　　　体重_____公斤

6. 孩子母亲现在的身高_____厘米　　　　体重_____公斤

7. 请根据您的判断，选择现阶段你们全家人的肥胖程度。

| 家庭成员 | 很瘦 | 有点瘦 | 正常体重 | 有点超重 | 严重超重 | 不能回答 |
|---|---|---|---|---|---|---|
| 孩子（指参加本次调查的孩子） | ☐ | ☐ | ☐ | ☐ | ☐ | ○ |
| 孩子的妈妈 | ☐ | ☐ | ☐ | ☐ | ☐ | ○ |
| 孩子的爸爸 | ☐ | ☐ | ☐ | ☐ | ☐ | ○ |
| 孩子的爷爷 | ☐ | ☐ | ☐ | ☐ | ☐ | ○ |
| 孩子的奶奶 | ☐ | ☐ | ☐ | ☐ | ☐ | ○ |
| 孩子的外公 | ☐ | ☐ | ☐ | ☐ | ☐ | ○ |
| 孩子的外婆 | ☐ | ☐ | ☐ | ☐ | ☐ | ○ |

8. 您的孩子是否曾患过可能导致肥胖的疾病（如糖尿病等内分泌类疾病）或曾经服用过可能导致肥胖的药物（如：糖皮质激素、胰岛素等激素类药物）？

☐ 1. 没有　　☐ 2. 有，请列出疾病或服用药物的名称_____

9. 孩子母亲的教育程度

☐ 小学或以下　☐ 初中　☐ 高中/中专　☐ 大专　☐ 本科　☐ 研究生或以上

10. 孩子父亲的教育程度

☐ 小学或以下　☐ 初中　☐ 高中/中专　☐ 大专　☐ 本科　☐ 研究生或以上

11. 您全家的<u>家庭月收入</u>（包括所有家庭成员的薪金收入、投资收入等）大约是多少？

□ 1500 元及以下　□ 1501－3000 元　□ 3001－6000 元
□ 6001－10000 元　□ 10001－20000 元　□ 20001－50000 元
□ 50001 元及以上

12. 平时您的孩子主要由谁照顾?

□ 我和丈夫（太太）　□ 孩子的爷爷奶奶或外公外婆
□ 保姆　□ 其他

13. 您家里人每周看电视，玩电脑游戏或上网加起来时间有多少?

孩子：_____小时/周　孩子父亲：_____小时/周　孩子母亲：_____小时/周

# CUHK 成年人闲暇运动量评级问卷

请您于下列 0－10 的等级中，**选取其中一个等级代表您过去一年内平均每星期的运动量**，然后填入下面方格中：（请参考下列附表中有关低强度、中等强度、及剧烈运动的例子）

**低强度运动**：是简单可以应付自如的运动，呼吸心跳没有明显加速，没有出汗。

**中等强度运动**：做这类运动时，呼吸和心跳稍微加快，轻微出汗，但不觉辛苦。

**剧烈运动**：做这类运动时，呼吸和心跳很快，大量出汗，觉得很辛苦。

从下表 **0－10 的等级中，只选一个等级填入此方格**───→ ☐

---

**没有运动习惯者，选 0 至 2**

0—完全没有任何运动，大部分时间是坐着或睡觉。

1—除了每次少于 10 分钟的慢步外，其余所有时间都没有运动。

2—除了每周一次少于 30 分钟的低强度运动外，其余所有时间都没有运动。

**平时有运动习惯者，选 3 至 6**

3—每星期都有一至两次 30 分钟以上低强度运动。

4—每星期都有三次以上 30 分钟以上低强度运动。

5—差不多每天都有一次 30 分钟以上低强度运动。

6—每星期都有一至两次 30 分钟以上中等强度运动。

**平时经常有运动习惯者，选 7 至 10**

7—每星期都有三次至五次中等强度运动（每次 30 分钟或以上）。

8—差不多每天都有中等强度运动（每次 30 分钟或以上）。

9—每星期都有不多于三次剧烈运动（每次 30 分钟或以上）。

10—差不多每天都有剧烈运动（每次 30 分钟或以上）。

---

**＊附表：低强度、中等强度、及剧烈运动的例子**

| | 低强度运动 | 中等运动 | 剧烈运动 |
|---|---|---|---|
| 体育运动 | 速度很慢的散步、遛狗 | 散步（健步行，速度较快）<br>慢跑 | 快速跑（感觉很辛苦） |
| | 保龄球 | 骑自行车 | 剧烈的篮球、足球比赛 |
| | 排球练习 | 投篮练习<br>嬉戏型式的游泳 | 连续游泳（不间断） |
| | 节奏较慢的舞蹈（如慢舞或华尔兹） | 舞蹈或健美操（低冲击性的健美操） | 越野跑步、定向越野 |
| | 玩飞碟 | 羽毛球练习 | |
| 家居活动 | 下楼梯 | 上下楼梯（混合） | 搬运大型东西或家具上楼梯 |
| | 逛街（较轻松、速度较慢、没有携带大量物品） | 用手或跪地型式的抹地；较辛苦的家务，如抹窗或洗车 | 剧烈的运动（如：连续做俯卧撑） |
| | 做比较轻松的家务，如抹地吸尘或清洁家居 | 家中的运动，如柔软体操、仰卧起坐等 | |
| | 站立或轻量的玩耍 | 携带不超过15斤物品步行上楼梯 | |
| | 在家中行走及搬动轻的物品 | 在游乐场游玩（有一定体力消耗的项目） | |
| | 弹吉他或其他乐器（站立） | | |

第二部分：请选择与您想法和行动一致的表述，并在相应的"□"内打"√"。

1. 我会关注我的孩子吃甜食的数量（如蛋糕、糖果、冰淇淋）

□从不　□很少　□有时　□经常　□总是

2. 我会关注我的孩子吃高脂食品的数量（如：油炸、膨化食品）

□从不　□很少　□有时　□经常　□总是

3. 我会关注我的孩子吃蔬菜水果的数量

□从不　□很少　□有时　□经常　□总是

4. 我的孩子吃零食之前要经过我同意

□从不　□很少　□有时　□经常　□总是

5. 我会关注我的孩子看电视、玩电子游戏、上网的时间

□从不　□很少　□有时　□经常　□总是

6. 我会关注我的孩子的体育锻炼的运动强度和时间

□从不　□很少　□有时　□经常　□总是

7. 假如我的孩子选择吃健康的食品，我会表扬他/她

□从不　□很少　□有时　□经常　□总是

8. 假如我的孩子积极参加体育运动，我会表扬他/她

□从不　□很少　□有时　□经常　□总是

9. 假如孩子表现好，我会给些零食（糖果，冰淇淋等）奖励他/她

□完全不同意　□不同意　□中立　□同意　□完全同意

10. 我应该特别关注，确保让我的孩子吃饱饭

□完全不同意　　□不同意　　□中立　　□同意　　□完全同意

11. 假如我的孩子说"我吃饱了"，我还是会尽量让他再吃一些

□完全不同意　　□不同意　　□中立　　□同意　　□完全同意

12. 假如我不对我孩子的饮食加以指导和调节，他就会吃得比他该吃的量少。

□完全不同意　　□不同意　　□中立　　□同意　　□完全同意

13. 假如孩子表现好，我会让他/她看电视或者玩电子游戏作为奖励。

□完全不同意　　□不同意　　□中立　　□同意　　□完全同意

14. 我会控制我的孩子喝含糖饮料的量（可乐，雪碧，鲜橙多等）

□完全不同意　　□不同意　　□中立　　□同意　　□完全同意

15. 我会控制我的孩子吃零食的数量

□完全不同意　　□不同意　　□中立　　□同意　　□完全同意

16. 周一到周五，我会控制孩子看电视，玩电子游戏的时间。

□完全不同意　　□不同意　　□中立　　□同意　　□完全同意

17. 周末，我会控制孩子看电视，玩电子游戏的时间。

□完全不同意　　□不同意　　□中立　　□同意　　□完全同意

**非常感谢您的参与！请将此问卷交由子女带回学校交给班主任。**

# CONTENTS

# ABSTRACT

Childhood obesity is becoming a challenging issue in China. Parents not only play key roles in childhood obesity control but also in the etiology of childhood obesity. Parental obesity is a strong predictor for a childhood obesity persisting into adulthood, especially for young children. Parents provide foods or make food choices for their children, which determine children's energy intake. In addition, parents can serve as role models and authority figures who not only help mold and shape dietary and physical activity habits in children but also influence children's attitudes and beliefs towards eating practices and sports participation. However, the relationships between certain parent-related factors and the development of adolescent obesity are rarely reported in China. Therefore, this study aims to investigate the relationship among Chinese parents' perception of their children's weight, parenting behaviors, parenting style, and adolescents' weight status. Two studies were performed to achieve this purpose.

The first study (Chapter 3) examines the validity and reliability of the questionnaires for adolescents and parents; the questionnaires are intended to measure parenting behaviors, parents' perception of their children's weight, and parenting styles in the Chinese context. Several steps were performed. First, the questionnaires were selected based on their validity and reliability, as well as their applicability to the Chinese adolescent and parenting context. Second, the questionnaires were translated into Chinese using a cross-cultural translation technique. Third, five experts were invited to evaluate the content validity and feasibility of the questionnaires for application in the Chinese population. Fourth, 15 pairs of adolescents and their parents were invited to attend a short interview after completing the experimental version of the questionnaires. They were asked to share comments on the readability and cultural relevance of the questionnaire. The questionnaires were then revised according to their feedbacks. Fifth, 127 pairs of adolescents (10 – 15 years old) and their parents (Ganzhou: 62 pairs, Shantou: 65 pairs) were recruited to examine the retest reliability and internal consistency of the questionnaires. Sixth, the data collected in the main survey were used to examine construct validity. The result showed that 10 items were excluded because of poor content validity or low intraclass correlation coefficient ( $< 0.7$ ). The internal consistencies of the subscales ( ranging from 0. 61 to 0. 81) were found to be acceptable ( Cronbach's $\alpha > 0.6$ ). The goodness-of-fit statistics ( RMSEA, CFI, and NNFI) also indicated acceptable fit for the theory models. The results suggest that the validity and reliability of the questionnaires are acceptable, and the questionnaires are applicable to Chinese adolescents and parents in Southern China.

The second study ( Chapters 4, 5, 6) determines the relationships among parenting behaviors, parents' perception of their children's weight, parenting style, and adolescent weight status. A total of 2, 143 adolescents and 1, 869 parents were recruited from secondary schools in Ganzhou and Shantou in China. The adolescents' weights and heights were measured by trained testers. The dietary habits and physical activity level of the adolescents, as well as parenting behaviors, parenting styles, parents' perception of their children's weight, and demographic information were collected through questionnaires issued to the adolescents and parents validated in Study 1. Several parenting behaviors, including "pressure to eat" and "diet and PA monitoring," were found to be significantly related to adolescents' age and gender-specific BMI Z score ( Z-BMI), although the correlation coefficients were low ( r ranged from $-0.23$ to 0. 09, $p < 0.01$). The results of the hierarchical multiple regression revealed that "pressure to eat" and "diet and PA monitoring" were the predictors of adolescent Z – BMI. The results of Kappa statistics showed that only a slight agreement exists between parental perception of their children's weights and the adolescents' actual weights ( Kappa = 0. 221, $p < 0.01$ ). A significant difference in parenting behaviors was found between parents with correct and incorrect perceptions of their children's weight. Parenting style could moderate the relation between adolescents' dietary habits, physical activity, weight status and parenting behaviors. The positive relation between parenting behavior of "restricting access to unhealthy food and youth's sedentary behaviors" and adolescents' dietary habits was alleviated as parents' reponsiveness increased. Furthermore, parents' demandingness moderated the effects of "food and physical activity monitoring" on adolescents' physical activity and weight status. The data of this study suggest that parenting behaviors are weakly but significantly associated with the development of adolescent obesity. Misclassifications of children's weight status are prevalent among Chinese parents. Parental perceptions of their children's weights are associated with some parenting behaviors related to children's weight development. The adolescents' dietary habits, physical activity, and some parenting behaviors are associated with parenting style. However, there is no direct association between parenting style and adolescent weight.

**Key words**: adolescent obesity, parenting behaviors, parenting styles

# ACKNOWLEDGEMENT

First and foremost, I would like to express my deep gratitude to my supervisor Prof. Stanley Sai Chuen Hui for his guidance, inspiration, understanding and patience during my Ph. D study in The Chinese University of Hong Kong. His continuous encouragement and generous support motivated me to keep optimistic and overcome adversities in my study and my life. The knowledge, courage and perseverance in academic and real life he shared with me will benefit me for a lifetime.

My sincere appreciations go to my thesis committee member Prof. Amy Sau Ching Ha and Prof. Stephen Heung Sang Wong for their invaluable advice and generous help. Thank you for your constructive suggestions and comments that enlighten my thoughts, opened my minds and led to a greatly improved thesis.

I am heartily thankful to my external examiner Prof. Pauline Po-lin Sung Chan for her valuable advice and generous help to my doctorial research, especially in the development of questionnaire and thesis revision.

I would like to thank Mr. Zheng yubin, Ms. Xie xiaofei, Mr. Yang ruilin, Mr. Xie peikai from Shantou University Medical College for their voluntary help in collecting data and data input. I also would like to extend my appreciation to all the participated adolescents, their parents and the school teachers who kindly helped me arranged the investigation.

Special thanks go to my colleagues and friends: Dr. Chen yajun, Dr. Wendy Huang Yajun, Mr. Wang Lin, Ms. Wang Lijuan, Mr. Sun Fenghua, Ms. Qi jing, Mr. He gang and Ms. Kiwi Chan. Their advice, encouragement and support in multiple ways made my life in CU a pleasant and memorable journey.

My warmest appreciation goes to my parents and wife for their unconditional support and love along the way. Thank you for listening to my complaints and frustrations, and for believing in me! No matter what happens, they are always there for me! For them, I dedicate this book.

# PUBLICATIONS

The findings presented in this thesis have been reported, in part, in the following publication and presentations.

**Wen, X.**, Hui SC. Chinese Parents' Perceptions of their Children's Weights and their Relation to Parenting Behaviors. *Child: Care, Health, Development.* 2011, 37 (3): 343 – 351. (SSCI)

**Wen, X.**, Hui SC. Parenting Style as a Moderator of Association Between Parenting Behaviors and Adolescent's Weight Status. *The Journal of Early Adolescence.* 2012 32: 252 – 268. (SSCI)

**Wen, X.** and Hui, S. C. Is parenting style associated to adolescent's physical activity? A cross-sectional study in southern China. *Paper presented at the American College of Sports Medicine's 57 Annual Meeting and World Congress on Exercise is Medicine*, Baltimore, The United States, June 1 – 5, 2010.

# ABBREVIATIONS

| | |
|---|---|
| AEE | Energy expenditure in physical activity |
| BMI | Body mass index |
| CFA | Confirmatory factor analysis |
| CFI | Comparative fit index |
| CI | Confidence interval |
| CVD | Cardiovascular disease |
| EE | Energy expenditure |
| NNFI | Non-normed fit index |
| PA | Physical activity |
| REE | Resting energy expenditure |
| RMSEA | Root mean square error of approximation |
| SES | Socioeconomic status |
| TEE | Total energy expenditure |
| TEF | Thermic effect of food |
| Z-BMI | Age and gender specific body mass index Z score |

# CHAPTER 1　INTRODUCTION

## 1.1　Background

During the past decades, childhood obesity became one of the worldwide public health problems. It is estimated that one out of ten school-aged children in the world were overweight (Lobstein, Baur, & Uauy, 2004). In Hong Kong , the prevalence of childhood obesity had increased closed to 70% from 1994 to 2007 (Yeung & Hui, 2007). From 1989 to 1997, the prevalence of obesity in urban area of China increased from 1.5% to 12.6%, and the prevalence of overweight increased from 14.6% to 28.6% (Luo & Hu, 2002).

As the prevalence of obesity is still growing and pediatric obesity increases the risk for adult obesity and numerous associated diseases (Choudhary, Donnelly, Racadio, & Strife, 2007; Gunnell, Frankel, Nanchahal, Peters, & Davey Smith, 1998), thousands of studies were done to find out the causes and appropriate treatments for the childhood obesity. Among these studies, two interesting phenomenon were discovered. First, children of obese parents seems to have higher risk for developing obesity (Treuth, Butte, & Sorkin, 2003). Second, parental involvement is related to weight loss in children (McLean, Griffin, Toney, & Hardeman, 2003). These studies indicated that parents may play important roles in the etiology and prevention of childhood obesity.

Obesity is the result of a long-term positive energy balance, which could be caused by multiple reasons (Barlow & the Expert Committee, 2007). Several possible risk factors for childhood obesity had been found, including lack of physical activity (Rennie, et al. , 2005), long television viewing time (Danner,

2008), a high consumption of fast foods (Bowman, Gortmaker, Ebbeling, Pereira, & Ludwig, 2004) and so on. Obviously, parents could be associated with most of these factors and can potentially mediate or buffer the impact of many of these factors. Parents were found to not only play key roles in children's behaviors formation but also have an effect on the development of children's food preference and dietary habits (Rhee, 2008). Furthermore, it was found that parents' feeding strategies (Faith, Berkowitz, et al., 2004) and parents' own food intake (Fisher, Mitchell, Wright, & Birch, 2002) could influence children's food intake. In addition, parental support (Prochaska, Rodgers, & James, 2002) and parents' own physical activity (Yang, Telama, & Laakso, 1996) were also found to be associated with their children's weight status. These studies suggested that parents could influence children's weight status through parenting behaviors.

As parenting behaviors is found to be influential in determining childhood obesity, the first question is what could motivate parents to choose or modify their parenting behaviors? Parents' readiness and willingness to modify their parenting behaviors may be one of the important steps in preventing childhood obesity. Recent study suggested that parental perception of children's weights could be associated with the parents' readiness to help their children lose weight (Rhee, De Lago, Arscott-Mills, Mehta, & Davis, 2005). Unfortunately, high percentages of parental misconception of their children's weight were reported in recent studies (Eckstein, et al., 2006; Etelson, Brand, Patrick, & Shirali, 2003; Ward, 2008). However, whether the parents' misconception of their children weight is associated with their parenting behaviors and the development of childhood obesity was not well reported.

Parenting behaviors is regarded as what parents do, while parenting style means how parents do it. Parenting style provides the emotional background how parenting behaviors are expressed and understood by children (Rhee, 2008). Parenting style was also found to be associated with childhood obesity. For example, parental neglect during childhood was found to predict a great risk of obesity in young adulthood, independent of age, gender, BMI in childhood, and social background ( Lissau & Sørensen, 1994 ). Another study showed that, compared to the children with authoritative mothers, children raised by authoritarian mothers had an higher risk of being overweight ( Rhee, Lumeng, Appugliese, Kaciroti, & Bradley, 2006 ). Therefore, childhood obesity intervention programs that include both parenting behaviors and parenting style may be more effective in weight loss and weight control than the traditional programs only focusing on behaviors ( Rhee, et al. , 2006).

Parenting behaviors and parenting style could be influenced by cultural difference. In China, traditional Chinese education is dominated by Confucianism for more than 2000 years. In traditional Chinese family, there is a strong bond between parents and children, and parent always play an extremely important role in determining their child's lifestyle. Even today, although Chinese society has been influenced by the West, many Chinese parents' beliefs and behaviors are still greatly influenced by Confucianism ( Holroyd, 2003; P. Wu, et al. , 2002; Xu, et al. , 2005 ). Chinese parenting was characterized by " restrictive ", "controlling" and "authoritarian" ( Lin & Fu, 1990; Steinberg, Dornbusch, & Brown, 1992). Research indicated that, Americans emphasize "nurturing innate ability" but Chinese attached great importance to high self-discipline, obedience to parents, which is one of the important parts in Chinese culture ( Chao, 1994; F. M. Chen & Luster, 2002). However, only several studies had investigated the association between the parenting behaviors, parenting style and their children's weight status in China. For example, a study based on 163 Chinese children and their mothers in Taiwan and United States showed that democratic parenting style is one of the factors that related to Chinese children's weight status ( J. L. Chen & Kennedy, 2004). Another study in Hong Kong found that parents may influence overweight children's attraction to physical activity ( Lau, Lee, & Ransdell, 2007).

Although several studies had been done on the influence of parenting behaviors and parenting styles on children's weight status in China, there are still many research questions that are not well answered. For instance, during the past 3 decades, the implementation of the single-child family planning program in the 1970s in mainland China not only caused a drastic decline in the natural growth rate of population in China (Jing, 1994), but could also influence millions of Chinese's parenting behaviors and parenting style. Many Chinese children are treated like a little emperor or empress at home by their parents, which could be significantly different from traditional Chinese parenting style. In addition, for hundreds years, the roles of mothers and fathers in China are quite different (Berndt, Cheung, Lau, Hau, & Lew, 1993), which indicated that, in China, the parenting behaviors and parenting style could also be different in mothers and fathers. However, little is known whether this gender difference in parenting is associated with children's weight status or not. Therefore, more studies are still needed to investigate the relationship among parenting behaviors, parents' perception of their children' weight, parenting styles and adolescents' weight status in China.

Furthermore, although a number of questionnaire and scales were developed to measure parenting behaviors and parenting styles (Birch, et al., 2001; Golan & Weizman, 1998; Hughes, Power, Fisher, Mueller, & Nicklas, 2003), most research regarding parenting behaviors and childhood obesity had been narrowly concentrated on a single aspect: parental control (Hughes, O'Connor, & Power, 2008). For example, Child Feeding Questionnaire (CFQ) is a frequently used instrument to measure parents' feeding beliefs, attitudes and behaviors. However, the confirmatory factor analysis showed that four out of seven factors in CFQ were focused on parental control practices (Birch, et al., 2001). In addition, because of the cultural difference, the questionnaire developed in western countries could not be directly applied in Chinese population without validity and reliability test.

In general, there are several research problems remained unsolved. First, few questionnaires are available to measure Chinese parents' parenting behaviors, parenting style and parents' perception of their children's weight. Second, the relationship among parenting behaviors, parenting style and parents' perception of their children's weight and children's weight status are still not clear. Third, limited data was reported on Chinese parenting behaviors, parenting style and parents' perception of their children's weight. Therefore, several research questions are proposed for the current study. First, is parenting behaviors associated with the development of adolescent obesity in China? Which parenting behaviors were associated with adolescent obesity? Second, is misperception of children's weight status prevalent in Chinese parents? Is parents' perception of their children's weight associated with their parenting behaviors? Third, is parenting style related to adolescent obesity? Is there any difference in parenting behaviors for the parents with different types of parenting style?

## 1.2  Purposes

Given the lack of questionnaires and studies on the association among Chinese parents' perception of their children's weight, parenting behaviors, parenting styles and adolescents' weight status, the purposes of this study are: 1) to examine the validity and reliability of questionnaires to measure Chinese's parenting behaviors, parents' perception of their children's weight and parenting styles; 2) to determine the relationship among adolescent weight status, parents' perception of their children's weight, parenting behaviors and parenting styles in China.

## 1.3  Significance

The significance of this study are summarized as follows: 1) The validated questionnaire in this study would be a valuable tool for practitioners and researchers for future evaluation and investigation; 2) Benefits parents with regards to effective parental style and behavior for combating obesity of their child; 3) Provides important information for designing effective strategies with regards to childhood obesity control; 4) Offers meaningful implications for policy makers for designing national health policy.

## 1.4  Hypotheses

**The null hypotheses are set as:**

I. The test-retest reliability, internal consistency and construct validity of the

216

questionnaires for adolescents and parents would not be satisfactory.

II. There is no agreement between the parents' perception of their children' weight status and the adolescents' actual weight status.

III. There is no association between parenting behaviors and adolescents' weight status.

IV. There is no association between parenting styles and their adolescents' weight status.

## 1.5    Operational definitions

### 1.5.1    Parents' perception of their children's weight status

In the present study, parents' perception of their children is defined as the self-reported parents' recognition and discrimination of their children's heaviness (Warschburger & Kroller, 2009).

### 1.5.2    Parenting behavior

In the current study, parenting behavior is defined as the parents' actions or reactions, which may influence their children's weight status, including parents' feeding strategies, parents' actions towards children's physical activity and sedentary behaviors (Rhee, 2008).

### 1.5.3    Parenting style

In the present study, parenting style is defined as the general mode of parenting reported by their children, which provides the emotional background how parenting behaviors are expressed and interpreted by adolescents (Darling & Steinberg, 1993).

### 1.5.4    Adolescent obesity

In this study, adolescent obesity is defined as body mass index (BMI) higher than the age and gender specific cutoff points based on the international growth standards for school-aged children and adolescents (Butte, Garza, & de Onis, 2007; De Onis, et al. , 2007).

## 1. 6　Limitations

First of all, as it is a cross-sectional study to determine the association between parenting behaviors, parenting styles and childhood obesity among Chinese, no information on causality relationship can be provided. Secondly, most of the data collected in the current study is based on participants' self-report. However, sometimes self-reported data may reflect participants' idealizations of themselves rather than actual realities. And sometimes participants would like to give the responses which are more socially acceptable.

## 1. 7　Delimitations

Firstly, due to vast territory in China and much higher prevalence of childhood obesity in urban regions as compared with in rural regions in China, the participants in this study were only recruited in two cities in southern China. In addition, only the grade one and grade two students in secondary schools were recruited in this study. Therefore, the findings of the study should be cautiously generalized to other age groups of children and parents as well as the children and parents in other locations.

Secondly, BMI rather than percent body fat was used to determine adolescents' and their parents' weight status. As BMI is not a direct indicator of body composition, sometimes high BMI is not equal to high percent body fat.

Thirdly, children and parents recruited for reliability test for questionnaire are ignorant of arrangement in repeated completion of the same questionnaire when they firstly are introduced to the study.

# CHAPTER 2   LITERATURE REVIEW

## 2. 1   Introduction

As obesity in children may lead to adult obesity and may increase the risk of chronic disease in adults, intervention programs for childhood obesity are urgently needed in order to control the development of obesity in adult population ( Magarey, Daniels, Boulton, & Cockington, 2003; Must & Strauss, 1999 ). However, most intervention programs for childhood obesity are characterized by patient non-attendance, high drop-out rate, and failure in weight maintenance ( Stewart, Chapple, Hughes, Poustie, & Reilly, 2008 ). Therefore, some new intervention programs resulting in long-term, sustained involvement in obesity control are still needed.

Recommendations from expert committee on childhood obesity pointed out the importance of parents' involvement in intervention ( Barlow & the Expert Committee, 2007 ). Some experts suggested the programs for childhood obesity should be family based with the participation of at least one parent, or it may lead to failure in treatment ( Dietz & Robinson, 2005; Robinson, 1999 ). Therefore, family based intervention, or even parents focused intervention could be an ideal long-lasting program for childhood obesity. One of the strong evidences of parents participation in obesity prevention is the study done by Epstein et al. , in which ten years effectiveness of a combined parent-child intervention program was demonstrated ( Epstein, Valoski, Wing, & McCurley, 1990 ).

Parents not only play key roles in treatment of childhood obesity but also in the etiology of childhood obesity. Parental obesity is a strong predictor for a childhood obesity persisting into adulthood, especially for young children (Whitaker, Wright, Pepe, Seidel, & Dietz, 1997). Parents provide foods or make food choices for their children. In addition, parents can serve as role models and authority figures who not only help mold and shape dietary and physical activity habits in children but also influence children's attitudes and beliefs towards eating practices and sports participation (Rhee, 2008).

Several literature reviews demonstrated the association between parental perceptions, parenting behaviors, parenting style, some other parent related factors and childhood obesity (Faith, Scanlon, Birch, Francis, & Sherry, 2004; Howard, 2007; Lindsay, Sussner, Kim, & Gortmaker, 2006; Rhee, 2008). However, although parental influence on childhood obesity is multi-factorial, majority of these studies only reviewed one or two factors. In addition, few studies focused on Chinese children and parents were included in these reviews. Therefore, in order to better understand the relationship between parents and childhood obesity, this review attempts to summarize the studies in recent years on the association between childhood obesity and some parents related factors, which include heredity, parental perception of their children's weight, parents' beliefs and knowledge on nutrition and obesity, parenting behaviors, parenting style, home environment, and some other related factors.

## 2. 2　Heredity and childhood obesity

The dramatic increase in the prevalence of childhood obesity in the past a few years was always reported to be associated with the changes in the environment (Franzini, et al., 2009; Strauss & Knight, 1999). However, not all children are influenced equally by unhealthy lifestyles. Some children remain lean even in a strongly obesogenic environment. There are really only two basic explanations for how these children keep lean (O'Rahilly & Farooqi, 2008). One is that the parents of these children always made right decision on their children's diet and exercise. Another reason is heredity. These lean children maybe somehow biologically different from other children and keep their weight status largely through some specific mechanisms.

## 2.2.1 Genetic influence on childhood obesity

### 2.2.1.1 Parent-offspring design studies

A recent study (Toschke, von Kries, Beyerlein, & Ruckinger, 2008) based on the data of 4, 884 children proved that maternal overweight could influence the entire BMI-distribution with an accentuation on upper quantiles to higher BMI values. However, some other factors including low meal frequency, formula feeding, maternal smoking in pregnancy, parental education, and high TV consumption could only leaded to a shift of upper quantiles. The data of another study suggested that, parents' weight status, birth BMI were independent predictors of children's BMI ( $r = 0.42$, $P < 0.001$ ) ( Schaefer-Graf, et al. , 2005). Another longitudinal study revealed that fathers' total or percentage body fat could predict their girls' long-term changes in total fat mass and percentage body fat ( Figueroa-Colon, Arani, Goran, & Weinsier, 2000). In addition, the data of another study showed parents'standardized weight change was significantly associated with children's standardized weight change for the 0 – to 6 – month ( $P < 0.001$) and 0 – to 24 – month ( $P < 0.009$) time points ( Wrotniak, Epstein, Paluch, & Roemmich, 2004). This study indicates that there is a link between children's weight and parents'. Children may get benefits from their parents who successfully lose weight in family-based intervention.

Similar results were also reported in China. A cross sectional survey based on 9, 325 children aged 6 – 8 in China showed that the prevalence of obesity in the children of normal weight parents was 11.1%. However, the prevalence of obesity in the children of obese parents was as high as 33.6% ( Y. Yu, Li, Xia, Tong, & Sun, 2002). The data of 2002 China National Nutrition and Health Survey, which included 6, 826 Chinese children aged 7 – 17 years, suggested that the heavier the parents' body weight, the higher risk for overweight in their children ( Y. Li, et al. , 2007). Another survey which investigated 11, 454 children aged 0 – 6 years in Shenzhen, showed that 13 factors are associated with childhood obesity, including parental overweight, father's low education, birth weight no less than four kilograms and some other factors ( B. Chen, et al. , 2008). These large sample investigations successfully demonstrated a significant association between childhood obesity and parental weight status in Chinese population.

It was suggested that increasing body fat in young women lead to intrauterine environments that, stimulate increased obesity among their children, generating an intergenerational acceleration of obesity levels ( Levin, 2000 ). If this mechanism is true, the correlation coefficient between maternal BMI and offspring BMI should be stronger than the correlation coefficient between father's BMI and their children's BMI. However, no significant difference was found between maternal-offspring and paternal-offspring BMI in 4, 654 families ( Smith, Steer, Leary, & Ness, 2007 ). Further studies are needed to determine whether children's weight status would be influenced by intrauterine environment.

### 2. 2. 1. 2　Twin design studies

The classical twin design is one of the most efficient measures in determining the contribution of shared genes and shared environment to familial traits. Compared with the parent-offspring design studies, the advantage of this design is providing a unique method for differentiating nature and nurture through the fact that monozygotic ( MZ ) twins share all of their genes, whereas dizygotic ( DZ ) twins share only half of their genes ( Hopper, Bishop, & Easton, 2005 ). According to the data of over 25, 000 twin pairs and 50, 000 biological and adoptive family members in published twin and adoption studies, it was summarized that the weighted mean correlations were 0. 74 for MZ twins, 0. 32 for DZ twins, 0. 25 for siblings, 0. 19 for parent-offspring pairs, 0. 06 for adoptive relatives, and 0. 12 for spouses ( Maes, Neale, & Eaves, 1997 ). Another studies measured the total and regional fat distribution of twins by DEXA ( Dual energy X-ray absorptiometry ) ( Malis, et al. , 2005 ). The results also showed that the intraclass correlations were higher for all fat percentages among MZ twins as compared with DZ twins. These studies suggested that genetic factors play an important role in variation of body fatness.

For the percentage of the fat mass that could be explained by gene, most studies reached similar conclusion, in which the heritability estimated in adults is about 55% to 86% ( Fabsitz, Sholinsky, & Carmelli, 1994; Faith, et al. ,

1999 ). For instance, a bivariate twin modeling was used to determine the contribution of the genetic factors to obesity, in which substantial heritability for obesity was found to be 0. 86 ( 95% CI, 0. 77 – 0. 94 ) ( Bulik, Sullivan, & Kendler, 2003 ). A recent study based on the data of BMI and waist circumference ( WC ) of more than five thousands twin pairs in United Kingdom confirmed that the substantial heritability for BMI and WC were both 77% ( Wardle, Carnell, Haworth, & Plomin, 2008 ). These studies support the importance of genes to the development of obesity.

### 2. 2. 1. 3　Limitations

One of the limitations in the parent-offspring or twin design studies is parent-offspring and sibling correlations do not separate the genetic and environmental transmission. Heritability could be overestimated in parent-offspring and twin studies as the family members share not only genetic but also the environmental factors. One solution for the shared environment problems in the parent-offspring or twin design studies is to choose the adoption study design. The logic of the adoption method is that resemblance in the trait between the adoptee and the biological family members could be explained by shared genes. However, resemblance between the adoptee and the adoptive family members should be shared family environment. For instance, based on 540 adult adoptees, some researchers had investigated the contributions of genetic factors and the family environment to percent body fat ( Stunkard, et al. , 1986 ), in which, a high correlation was found between the weight status of the adoptees and their biologic parents. However, no relation was found between the weight status of the adoptees and their adoptive parents.

Another limitation for parents-offspring design study is the heritability could be underestimated because children and parents are measured at different ages. If different genetic and/or environmental factors account for the variation in BMI at different ages, parent-offspring and sibling correlations would be reduced and heritability could be underestimated. In addition, variability in heritability estimate is very large due to different study design ( twin, family, and adoption studies ) , small sample and large variation in ages of participants ( Beunen, et al. , 1998 ). Although there are several limitations in these studies, parent-offspring and twin design studies are still effective and widely applied in genetic epidemiology. These studies had also successfully demonstrated that genetic factors are one of the most important factors in the etiology of childhood obesity.

## 2. 2. 2  Genetic influence on energy expenditure

An imbalance of energy intake relative to energy expenditure ( EE ) could lead to obesity. Possible mechanisms for the etiology of obesity, which is proved to be associated with genes, may include low energy expenditure and/or high energy intake ( Figueroa-Colon, et al. , 2000).

### 2. 2. 2. 1  Resting energy expenditure

50% to 75% of total energy expenditure of a person is spent as resting energy expenditure ( REE ) ( Ravussin & Bogardus, 1989 ). Interindividual difference in REE could be one of the causes for obesity. Some early studies showed that children of obese parents had low REE ( Griffiths & Payne, 1976; Griffiths, Payne, Stunkard, Rivers, & Cox, 1990), which could contribute to childhood obesity. It was reported that 11% of the variance in the REE may be explained by family membership ( Bogardus, et al. , 1986 ). The intraclass correlation coefficient for familial influence and energy expenditure, independent of percent body fat, age and gender was found to be 0. 26 ( Ravussin & Bogardus, 1989). Recent studies on REE and obesity showed that heritability of REE was 0. 30 after body size were controlled ( X. Wu, et al. , 2004 ), and heritability was 0. 29 ± 0. 08 for REE after thyroid hormones and metabolic risk were adjusted ( Bosy-Westphal, et al. , 2008).

However, the data of some studies did not support for the theory that the children of obese parents have low REE and therefore have higher odds for overweight. For example, prepubertal girls with either lean or obese parents were found to have similar EE during rest, sleep, some types of physical activity and over a 24-h period ( Treuth, Butte, & Wong, 2000). The results of another study showed that, compared with the children of nonobese parents, the adjusted mean REE was 50 kcal/day lower in children when only the mother was obese or only the father was obese, but not when both parents were obese ( Goran, et al. ,

1995). Some researchers pointed out that one reason for the undiscovered relation between low metabolic rate and overweight could be that obesity-related metabolic risk factors mask the problem of low metabolic rate which may initially lead to overweight (Bosy-Westphal, et al., 2008).

### 2. 2. 2. 2　Thermic effects of food

The thermic effect of food (TEF) is the increase in energy expenditure after food intake. TEF was investigated for decades. However, it is still not clear whether TEF contribute to the development of obesity. The heritability of TEF was reported by only a couple of studies. The data of a study showed that at least 40% to 50% of the variation of TEF could be explained by genes. The correlations for TEF in DZ, MZ and parent-spring pairs were 0. 35, 0. 52 and 0. 30 respectively (Bouchard, et al., 1989). In another study, TEF during exercise, was found to be significantly higher for the normal men when compared with obese men in submaximal intensities exercise (Segal, Presta, & Gutin, 1984). These studies suggested that the children of obese parents are more likely to have a low TEF, which may make them more likely to increase weight.

### 2. 2. 2. 3　Activity related energy expenditure and total energy expenditure

Energy expenditure in physical activity (AEE) is an key component of the total energy expenditure (TEE). Several studies suggested that the interindividual differences in AEE and TEE could be partly explained by heredity. For instance, it was found out that reduced energy expenditure, particularly on physical activity, play a key role in the rapid weight gain in infants born to overweight mothers (Roberts, Savage, Coward, Chew, & Lucas, 1988). Another study investigated the weight status and the energy expenditure of 196 nonobese girls, in which the data of REE and TEE were measure by indirect calorimetry and doubly labeled water method respectively. The data showed that TEE was found to be higher among girls with at least an overweight parent (Bandini, Must, Spadano, & Dietz, 2002). However, another study based on a large sample of healthy infants showed no aspect of infant energy expenditure was associated with parents' weight status (Davies, Wells, Fieldhouse, Day, & Lucas, 1995).

## 2. 2. 3    Genetic influence on energy intake and food preference

When energy intake is greater than energy expenditure, even at modest daily energy surpluses, could cause the problem of childhood obesity ( Goran, 2001 ). The result of an animal study suggested that the macronutrients consumption in the diet seems to be partly heritable ( Reed, Bachmanov, Beauchamp, Tordoff, & Price, 1997 ). Similar results were also found in the research on the development of children's dietary habits and food preference. It was found out that children were predisposed to reject unfamiliar foods and to learn the relation between foods' flavors and the post-ingestive consequences of eating ( Birch & Fisher, 1998 ). In addition, this study also showed that children could respond to the energy density of the diet, which indicated that children's energy intake and food selection may be influenced by their genes.

On the other hand, several twin studies were undertaken to determine the influence of heredity in energy intake and food preference. A study investigated 3-d dietary record in 1597 subjects living in 375 families of French descent ( Perusse, et al. , 1988 ). However, the results showed no significant genetic effect on any tested nutrient intake ( heritability $\leqslant 11\%$ ), which indicated that the genetic factor may not be the most important in children's food selection and that nongenetic effects maybe the major predictors of food intake. There are still some other studies indicated the presence of familial influence on energy intake and food preferences. For example, a study found that similarity among MZ twins exceeded that among DZ twins for intake of several types of food, which suggested that genes influence people's foods preferences ( Heitmann, Harris, Lissner, & Pedersen, 1999 ). Another classic twin design study based on 396 twin pairs also showed an evidence of genetic influences on children's food intake ( Faith, Rhea, Corley, & Hewitt, 2008 ).

In general, the results reviewed here suggest there is an association between food intake and genes. Although the heritability level may be not very high, there are increasing evidences that genes play an important role in energy intake and food preference, which has the potential to increase the risk for obesity.

## 2. 3 Parental perception, belief and knowledge of childhood obesity

Heredity is one of the factors influencing childhood obesity but maybe not a major factor in determining the development of childhood obesity ( Harrell, Bomar, McMurray, Bradley, & Deng, 2001 ). Studies showed that besides biological and developmental factors, a series of psychological, social, cultural, and environmental factors also influenced children's food consumption and physical activity (Sallis, et al. , 1992 ). For the parents who want to actively engage in obesity prevention, parental perception of children's weight status, health belief toward childhood obesity as well as their knowledge on nutrition and exercise could be very important in childhood obesity treatment.

### 2. 3. 1 Parental perception of children's weight status

Some studies had proved that adolescents typically underestimate their weight status ( Skinner, Weinberger, Mulvaney, Schlundt, & Rothman, 2008 ). Furthermore, it was found that the obese and overweight adolescents who had an accurate perception of weight were more likely to participate in weight-related behavior modification ( Bittner Fagan, Diamond, Myers, & Gill, 2008 ). A Portuguese study found incorrect perceptions of the need to diet, poorer self-perceived health status in the children with overweight ( Fonseca & Gaspar de Matos, 2005 ). However, one problem is whether parents could correctly classify the weight status of their children. Another problem is whether parents of overweight adolescents who recognize their children's weight problems are more likely to help their children control weight or not.

Unfortunately, most studies showed that parents always regarded their children' weight as less severe than it actually was ( Skinner, et al. , 2008 ). It was reported that nearly one third of mothers misperceive their overweight children as being lower than their actual weight status ( Maynard, Galuska, Blanck, & Serdula, 2003 ). A qualitative study revealed parents had a distorted view of clinically defined overweight preschoolers, and many of them did not regard overweight and obesity as health problems ( Suzanne Goodell, Pierce, Bravo, &

Ferris, 2008). It is also found that nearly all of the obese mothers classify themselves as overweight, but most of these mothers did not regard their overweight children as overweight. The study also revealed that mothers with less education were more likely to have misperception on their children's weight status (Baughcum, Chamberlin, Deeks, Powers, & Whitaker, 2000). Another study also suggested that few parents of overweight or "at risk of overweight" children classified their child as overweight or were worried about their child's overweight problem (Eckstein, et al. , 2006).

Therefore, the development of obesity prevention strategies and weight management programs may need to consider the issue of parental misperception of children's weight status. Moreover, some studies had suggested that the parents and children, who underestimated the children's weight, were more likely to have poorer diet behaviors and more obstacles for the adoption of healthy diet and physical activity behaviors (Skinner, et al. , 2008). A study had examined the psychological effects feedback to parents. During this study, the height and weight of children aged 6-11 years in London schools were tested, and parents were informed their children's weight status. Health behavior modification information was collected 6 weeks before and 4 weeks after the feedback which showed that feedback did not influence feeding behaviors in parents of healthy-weight children, but the application of food restriction strategies was increased among parents of overweight girls ( Grimmett, Croker, Carnell, & Wardle, 2008 ). However, another cross sectional study showed that accurate perception of child weight status may not lead to helpful behaviors but may cause unhealthy behaviors such as pressure to diet (Neumark-Sztainer, Wall, Story, & van den Berg, 2008). One of the possible reasons for these conflicting results in different studies could be the different research designs, especially in the intervention design. Additional randomized, controlled intervention studies were still needed to determine whether this kind of interventions were effective or not in children's weight management.

### 2. 3. 2　Parental belief and knowledge about nutrition and exercise

Four categories of factors were found to influence food consumption: consumer's income, food prices and prices of other products and service, consumer's tastes &

preference, and consumer's beliefs and knowledge of health and nutrition (Variyam & Blaylock, 1998). Therefore, it was believed that the parents with good nutrition knowledge were more likely to choose healthy food for their children. A survey from England showed that the subjects in the highest quintile for knowledge were almost 25 times more likely to meet the diet recommendations than those in the lowest quintile (Wardle, Parmenter, & Waller, 2000). In another study, mothers' nutritional knowledge and health diet-related beliefs were found to be important predictors of children's fruit intake (Gibson, Wardle, & Watts, 1998), fiber intakes and lower fat intakes (Variyam, Blaylock, Lin, Ralston, & Smallwood, 1999). In addition, mothers' awareness of diet and health relationships were also found to be associated with their teen children's dairy consumption, although mothers' health awareness did not influence preschool children and primary school children's dairy product consumption (Kim & Douthitt, 2003). The inconsistent results found in these findings suggested that nutrition knowledge may play a small but important role in the adoption of healthy dietary habits (Worsley, 2002).

Increasing children and adolescents' physical activity participation is one of the main objectives of childhood obesity prevention. Some studies had proved that exercise knowledge was one of the predictors for physical activity in both adults (Hagger, Chatzisarantis, & Biddle, 2002) and children (Trost, et al., 1997). For instance, the results of a longitudinal study suggested that prior knowledge predicted subsequent exercise behavior (Rimal, 2001). Another study also found that physical activity level could be associated with the knowledge of appropriate exercise intensity to keep health and the belief of exercise adherence (Fitgerald, Singleton, Neale, Prasad, & Hess, 1994). Therefore, parents' beliefs and knowledge on exercise could be indirect predictors of their children's physical activity. For example, it was found that parents who paid great attention to their children's physical activity were more likely to give their backing to their children's physical activity by, for instance, transporting them to sporting events et al. (Trost, et al., 2003). However, there was still study indicated that children's perceptions of their parents' beliefs were not associated with children's physical activity level ( Kimiecik, Horn, & Shurin, 1996 ). Another study also indicated that knowledge and attitudinal factors had far low correlation to obesity than activity-related behavioral factors ( Gordon-Larsen, 2001 ). Nevertheless, the results of most studies support including knowledge and beliefs in nutrition and exercise as one of the components for parents in childhood obesity prevention.

2.3.3　Chinese tradition and parental perception, beliefs and knowledge of obesity

Parental perception, beliefs and knowledge of obesity could be associated with cultural values. There are research evidences of ethnic and cultural difference in levels of body weight dissatisfaction and dieting behaviors ( Altabe, 1998; Gluck & Geliebter, 2002 ). In China, some Chinese traditional ideas on obesity and poor knowledge on nutrition and physical activity maybe associated with the increase prevalence of childhood obesity. For example, in Chinese traditional culture, obese children are always regarded as healthy children, and good appetite is always associated with health ( Y. N. Li, 2008 ). A study based on 140 obese children showed that 36% fathers and 28% mothers did not realized that their children were obese, and some parents even regard obesity as a characteristic of good health ( Xiao, Yang, & He, 2001 ). A survey on Chinese parents' knowledge on obesity showed that the parents of obese children got lower scores in the obesity knowledge test, when compared with the parents of normal weight children ( J. G. Wang, Cui, Su, & Wang, 2007 ). Another intervention study was conducted to improve parental perception and knowledge on obesity. The data of questionnaire survey before and after intervention showed that parental knowledge on diet could be improved by intervention ( Lv & Tian, 2007 ). One limitation for these studies was the sources or the procedure of questionnaire development was not clearly introduced. The reliability and validity of the questionnaires were not provided as well. Nevertheless, these studies still demonstrated that parental perception, belief and knowledge on obesity could be associated with childhood obesity in China.

China is famous for her refined art of the cooking skills in Chinese food preparation. However, in China, most people care about the color, fragrance, flavor and shape of food, but relatively less attention is paid to the nutrient component of food. Therefore, in Chinese family, it always the flavor of food rather than the nutrition or contained calories concerns parents ( Y. N. Li, 2008 ). In addition, many Chinese adults have an unforgettable poverty experience in their childhood, which increase their motivation to feed their children with abundant food. In a qualitative study, some Chinese reported that they experienced extreme hunger and destitution during 1940s to 1970s, and this miserable experience made them always worry that their children may not have enough food intake, and tend to provide young children with excessive food than they really need ( Jiang, et al. , 2007)

In Chinese tradition, children's academic performance at school is always a primary concern for Chinese parents. It is also noteworthy that education is one of the most important ways of personal advancement in mainland China ( Xiang, Lee, & Solmon, 1997 ). Therefore, any activities ( including physical activities ) that may negatively influence children's academic performance, maybe not supported by their parents. For instance, a study made an investigation on parents whose children were student players at track and field teams in middle schools. The results showed that, although most parents believed sports training is good for children's health and fitness, most parents still would not support their children to attend school team training, because the training would take up a lot of children's time and may have adverse affect on their children's academic performance ( C. L. Li & Li, 2005 ). Another study in Hong Kong also suggested that concepts associated with the intersection of Confucianism and postcolonialism will help to interpret the relatively subordinate place of sports and physical activity in the lives of Hong Kong families ( Ha, Macdonald, & Pang, 2010).

In summary, only a few studies investigated the parental perception, beliefs and knowledge on childhood obesity, diet and exercise in China. The results of these studies suggested that parental perception, beliefs and knowledge on obesity, diet and exercise could be influenced by Chinese traditional culture. Further studies are needed to promote healthy eating and sufficient physical activity in Chinese children.

## 2. 4　Parenting behavior

### 2. 4. 1　Parenting behavior and children's food intake

### 2. 4. 1. 1　Parental feeding behavior and children's food intake

Children's diet, which is one of the most important environmental factors in the etiology of childhood obesity (Birch & Fisher, 1998), could be influenced by parents, friends, school, the media and their own taste and preference (Golan & Crow, 2004a; Lindsay, et al. , 2006). A prominent parental influence on children's eating may be parents' feeding behaviors, which include restriction of food, pressure to eat, using food as a reward and other behaviors. Parental feeding behavior may influence the development of children's eating habits and food preference, their ability to regulate energy intake, and ultimately their weight status (Nguyen, Larson, Johnson, & Goran, 1996). A comprehensive literature review examined 22 studies on the association between parental feeding strategies, children's energy intake and weight status (Faith, Scanlon, et al. , 2004). The results showed that, although study methodologies and results could be different, nineteen studies (86%) reported at least one significant association between parental feeding behaviors and children's weight status. Therefore, parental feeding strategies could be important factors influencing the development of childhood obesity.

*Restricting Access to Food*

One of the most frequently used parental feeding behaviors toward childhood obesity is restriction of portion sizes or unhealthy food eaten. Parents who use this type of feeding behaviors may believe what they are doing is good for their child's health. However, this assumption was not approved by the data found in recent research. A observational study was taken to determine the effects of restricting access to a palatable food on children's food choice. It was found that compared with a similar snack food that was not restricted, children showed more interest to a restricted snack food after a 5-week period of restriction (Fisher & Birch,

1999b). The results based on a longitudinal study also showed that girls' dietary habit of eating snack foods in the absence of hunger could be predicted by parents' reports of restricting their daughter's access to foods (Fisher & Birch, 2002). Another longitudinal study also demonstrated that parents' restriction feeding strategies at age 5 predicted higher BMI at age 7, even when BMI at age 3 was adjusted for (Faith, Berkowitz, et al., 2004).

Possible mechanisms were proposed by several researchers to explain the association between parents' restriction feeding strategies and children's weight status. Restricting access may focus children's attention on restricted foods, while increasing their desire to get and eat those foods (Fisher & Birch, 1999b). Therefore, parents' restriction feeding strategy may decrease the intake of unhealthy food and total calories of a meal. However, children may try to obtain and consume the restricted food when they are out of parental control. An observational study supported this hypothesis (Klesges, Stein, Eck, Isbell, & Klesges, 1991). It was found that, when children were allowed to freely select foods from dozens of foods, they chose a large amount of unhealthy food of which nearly 25% of all kilocalories are in the form of added sugar. However, when they were informed that parent would be monitoring the meal they chose, children modified their food choices by decreasing their food selection or by selecting fewer unhealthy foods.

As considerable evidences for negative effects of restriction feeding strategy were provided, this feeding behavior should not be recommended for parents. Recent research recommended that information and guidance on feeding strategies and skills should be given to parents, particularly for the ones who cared about their child's weight (Clark, Goyder, Bissell, Blank, & Peters, 2007).

*Pressure to eat*

Another feeding behavior parents usually use is pressure to eat (prompting to eat or encouragement to eat), which means encourage children finish all the foods on their plate or force them to eat some types of food. Some studies had showed that this kind of feeding strategy may increase children's fruit and vegetable intake

(Bourcier, Bowen, Meischke, & Moinpour, 2003). Moreover, a study indicated that parents' "pressure to eat" strategy could be negatively related to children's total fat mass (Spruijt-Metz, Lindquist, Birch, Fisher, & Goran, 2002). Another study based the college students' memory showed that "pressure to eat" feeding strategy could lead to children's long-lasting negative feeling towards to that food (Batsell, Brown, Ansfield, & Paschall, 2002).

Further examination of the children's response to the feeding behavior of pressure to eat, may help us further understand the influence of "pressure to eat" on child weight status. It was found out that, young children of obese mothers were found to be more likely to use the strategy of "pressure to eat", especially for novel food, while children of nonobese mothers were not (Lumeng & Burke, 2006). Interestingly, the study also revealed that in the same study obese mothers also prompted their child more often when the food was novel than when it was familiar.

In general, the variability in these studies suggested that the relationship between "pressue to eat" and children's weight status may be more complicated than it appears. Encouraging or forcing children to eat some kind of food may increase this kind of food intake. However, in the long run, this strategy may lead to children's long-lasting negative feelings toward this food.

*Use food as rewards*

Using food to shape children's behaviors is also a common applied parental feeding behavior. An survey on the child-feeding practices of low-income mothers showed that, besides using food to provide energy and nutrient to their children, food was also frequently applied to promote good behaviors (Baughcum, Burklow, Deeks, Powers, & Whitaker, 1998). It was believed that, this kind of feeding behavior to promote good behaviors unassociated with hunger could disarrange children's ability to perceive their normal hunger and satiety cues. An experimental study indicated that presenting food as reward enhanced preference for that food (Birch, Zimmerman, & Hind, 1980). This sort of parenting behavior, if applied continuously, may cause long term adverse effects on a child's ability to self-regulate energy intake and lead to an increased reliance on external cues to determine how much to eat ( Rhee, 2008 ). Therefore, this kind of parenting behavior may lead children to get much more calories than they need.

There are several issues should be noticed in the studies on parenting behaviors and children's dietary habits. Firstly, several studies had revealed that the relationship between parental feeding behaviors and child's weight status is likely to be bi-directional, but cross-sectional studies could not determine the causes and effects relationship ( Clark, et al. , 2007; Faith, Berkowitz, et al. , 2004). For instance, parents may use restrict child access to unhealthy food, if the child are overweight. However, children could be lean just because their parents use this restriction strategy. It could be one of the possible reasons why association between parental feeding styles and children's weight status can not be found in some cross-sectional studies ( Baughcum, et al. , 1998; Saelens, Ernst, & Epstein, 2000).

Another factor that may influence the parental feeding behavior is socioeconomic status. In a qualitative study, some feeding beliefs and behaviors that may be associated with childhood obesity were found in some mothers with low socioeconomic status ( Baughcum, et al. , 1998). For instance, mothers with low socioeconomic status were found to be more likely to use food to shape their children's behaviors. Another study also showed that mothers with low education levels were more likely to use " pressure to eat" strategy ( Lumeng & Burke, 2006). Therefore, the results of these studies indicated that more studies are needed to identify interventions that are effective across different socioeconomic groups or design different programs for different groups.

In summary, various parental feeding behaviors were found to be involved in the etiology of childhood obesity. It was recommended that parent should let children to grow in a nature way, in which parents are responsible for the what, when and where of feeding, while children are responsible for the how much and whether of eating ( Satter, 2004).

### 2. 4. 1. 2   Parental modeling and children's food intake

Another parenting behavior that may have influence on children's dietary habits could be through role modeling or observational learning. A recent study in a laboratory setting indicated that children had higher odds to eat new food if others were eating the same kind of food than when others were only present or eating another kind of food ( Addessi, Galloway, Visalberghi, & Birch, 2005). Therefore, it was hypothesized that, by eating and drinking healthy foods and showing their children that they enjoy the food, parents may influence their children's dietary intake ( Golan & Crow, 2004a; Lindsay, et al. , 2006). Some studies proved this hypothesis. A statistically significant but modest correlation coefficient ( $r < 0.50$ ) was found between parents' and children's intake of many types of foods ( Oliveria, et al. , 1992). The frequency with which parents model healthful dietary behaviors were also found to have long-term influence on development of childhood eating habits ( Tibbs, et al. , 2001). In addition, another study demonstrated that parents' own fruit and vegetable intake may promote their daughters' fruit and vegetable intake, leading to higher micronutrient intakes and lower dietary fat intakes ( Fisher, et al. , 2002). When adolescents get older, they may also get increasingly support from their friends. However, it was found that families still play a continued key role in providing support to adolescents in the African-American families ( Wilson & Ampey-Thornhill, 2001). Through these studies, it is clear that parents can indirectly mold their children's behaviors through role modeling. Therefore, adoption of healthy behaviors is strongly recommended for parents in order to better modify their children's eating behaviors in children obesity intervention program.

## 2.4.2 Parenting behavior and children's physical activity level

Current guideline for children recommended at least 60 minutes of physical activity on most, preferably all, days of the week, however, currently most of the children can not meet the recommendation for 60 minutes of daily physical activity ( Nicklas, Hayes, & American Dietetic Association, 2008). Sport or physical activity participation is a very complex behavior which could be influenced by many factors. Schools have been regarded to play a central role in promoting physical activity in children and adolescents ( Pate, et al. , 2006). However, it is parent determine whether or not children could walk to school, how far they are allowed to ride bicycle, and facilitate attendance at out-of-school activities such as dancing and swimming. Therefore, parents also play key roles in children's physical activity participation (Mulvihill, Rivers, & Aggleton, 2000).

Parents could support their children to do physical activity in many forms. It could be in the form of payment of sportswear or sports shoes, driving children to playground, encouraging children to do physical activity or frequently doing exercise as a model (Prochaska, et al. , 2002). Research on parental influences helps determine several dimensions of parenting behaviors that could be important: acceptance and social support, role modeling, expressing expectations, reinforcing behavior by rewarding and punishing, controlling behavior and giving detailed instructions (Woolger & Power, 1993).

### 2. 4. 2. 1　Modeling

One of the most important parental behaviors influencing children's physical activity level could be role modeling. The data from Framingham Children's Study showed that children of physically active parents had significant higher odds ratio for being physically active when compared with the children of inactive parents. Moreover, when both parents were active, the children were 5. 8 times as likely to be active as children of two physically inactive parents (Moore, et al. , 1991). A survey in Norway also showed that adolescents' sport participation is influenced by their family members' and peers' sport participation, and part of the explanation for participation was based on the adolescent's relationship with physically active family members (Skille, 2005). These studies suggested that the one of the possible reasons for the association between parents' and children's physical activity levels could be parental role modeling. A recent qualitative study also suggested that parental role modeling is one of the most important factors to consider in designing programs for physical activity promotion among adolescents (Wright, Wilson, Griffin, & Evans, 2008). In general, these studies had clearly demonstrated that children's physical activity level could be influenced through parents' role modeling.

### 2. 4. 2. 2　Parent support

Several reviews had summarized the studies on parental support and children's physical activity ( Sallis, Prochaska, & Taylor, 2000; van der Horst, Paw, Twisk, & Van Mechelen, 2007 ). Unfortunately, the findings are still inconclusive. For example, some studies had found that the children with more parental support for sport participation were more active ( O'Loughlin, Paradis, Kishchuk, Barnett, & Renaud, 1999 ). Adolescents who received parental encouragement to exercise had significantly more physically active days in a week than did their counterparts ( King, Tergerson, & Wilson, 2008 ). However, it was also found that parental support was not a significantly factor associated with objectively measured physical activity level ( Sallis, Taylor, Dowda, Freedson, & Pate, 2002 ). It was reported that parent's reported support maybe related to girl's physical activity, although the correlation was not statistically significant ( $r = 0.26$, $p < 0.06$ ). However, it was found that the girl's reported of their parent's support for physical activity was not associated with girl's activity levels ( Adkins, Sherwood, Story, & Davis, 2004 ). Another study based on self-reported and accelerometer measured adolescents' physical activity level showed that parent support significantly correlated with adolescent self-reported physical activities. But the researchers failed to find significant association between parent support and adolescent's physical activity level measured by accelerometers ( Prochaska, et al. , 2002 ).

In summary, there are considerable inconsistent results in the studies on the association between parent support and children's physical activity level. Some possible explanations for this inconsistency could be the difference in the research methods measuring physical activity, sample characteristics and statistical analysis ( van der Horst, Paw, et al. , 2007 ). For example, physical activity level was determined by different questionnaires and objective measures ( such as accelerometer or pedometer ). Some studies recruited their young research participants with overweight or at risk of overweight, whereas populations of normal weight children were included in other studies. Therefore, additional studies are still needed to determine the relationship between parental support and children's physical activity level.

### 2. 4. 3　Parenting behaviors and childhood obesity in China

The research from western countries had proved the association between parenting behaviors and childhood obesity. Given that the social structure and traditional culture in China is different from them in western countries, it is plausible that the parenting behaviors in Chinese parents such as feeding behaviors and parental support to children's physical activity may be different.

"Pressure to eat" was reported to be one of the most common feeding strategies used by parents from western countries (Bourcier, et al. , 2003; Spruijt-Metz, et al. , 2002). The research indicated that this kind of feeding strategy is also frequently applied in Chinese parents. However, most Chinese parents just choose to remind rather than force their children to eat food. It was reported that 56. 0% parents often reminded their children to eat some food they regarded as healthy food, and 7. 7% parents often forced their children to eat these food (W. J. Ma, Du, Lin, Ren, & Ma, 2001). One parenting behavior that rarely reported in American or European parents but very common in China could be "criticize children during dinner". It was found that 14. 8% and 27. 5% of parents often or sometimes criticized their children during dinner, respectively, which could make 5. 9% children could not eat anything during the dinner (W. J. Ma, et al. , 2001). In addition, a cross sectional study based on 930 families with 2 – to 6 – year – old children in Beijing revealed a strong relation between parents' and children's dietary habits, TV watching and physical activity (Jiang, et al. , 2006).

Research in China also showed that parents may influence children's physical activity through role modeling and providing financial or emotional support (C. Sun, Zhang, Niu, & Ma, 2008). For example, a cross sectional study on 1, 614 middle school students in Hefei showed that the children of active parents were more likely to be physically active (Y. H. Sun, Be, & Ni, 1994). Another study from 104 parents of overweight children in Hong Kong showed that parental influence, especially father's role modeling, was significantly related to overweight Chinese children's physical activity participation (Lau, et al. , 2007).

Although some meaningful studies has been taken to investigate the influence of parenting behaviors on childhood obesity in China, there are still several limitations in these studies that needed to be acknowledged. For example, as parenting behaviors may be influenced by cultural factors, Chinese parents could have some unique parenting behaviors with Chinese characteristics. For instance, some parents always like to add some dishes to their children to express their love to children. This feeding strategy could influence children's own capability to regulate calories intake. However, the relationship between these traditional Chinese parenting behaviors and children's weight status was not well reported. Few studies investigated the differences in the parenting behaviors between Chinese parents and western parents. Nevertheless, these Chinese studies still successfully demonstrated that the parenting behaviors are associated with Chinese children's weight status.

## 2.5　Parenting style

Parenting behaviors or practices is regarded as what parents do, while parenting style is thought of how parents do it. Parenting style is defined as "the general pattern of parenting that provides the emotional background in which parent behaviors are expressed and interpreted by the child" (Rhee, 2008). Therefore, parenting style may not only influence parents' feeding strategies and behaviors towards children's physical activity, but may also influence children's physical activity activities, eating habits, emotional functioning, and ultimately the risk for overweight. Intervention that attaches importance to both parenting style and parenting behaviors could be more effective in childhood obesity prevention than present treatments only concentrated on parenting behaviors (Rhee, et al. , 2006).

### 2.5.1　The construct of parenting style

The most widely used typology was originally established by Baumrind, in which parenting styles were conceptualized based on the amount and quality of two underlying dimensions: demandingness and responsiveness (Baumrind, 1971). According to these two dimensions, parenting could be categorized into four main

styles: ( 1 ) the authoritative style ( high demandingness/high responsiveness )
( 2 ) the authoritarian style ( high demandingness/low responsiveness ) ; ( 3 ) the
indulgent/permissive style ( low demandingness/high responsiveness ) and ( 4 )
the uninvolved/neglectful style ( low demandingness/low responsiveness )
( Darling & Steinberg, 1993 ).

## 2. 5. 2    The influence of parenting style on children

The authoritative parenting style is considered to be the best parenting style
and was reported to be associated with improved child outcomes. In contrast, the
other three parenting style do not satisfy children's developmental needs, and
therefore has been associated with poorer outcomes among children. For example,
it was reported that parenting styles may influence adolescents' academic
achievement and performance ( Aunola, Stattin, & Nurmi, 2000 ). It was also
found that authoritative parents were found to be successful in keeping their
children from problem drug use ( Baumrind, 1991 ).

Some studies had also reported the association between the parenting style and
children's weight status. Data based on 4, 983 4 – to 5 – year – old children in the
first wave of the nationally representative Longitudinal Study of Australian
Children showed that, children of fathers with permissive and uninvolved parents
had higher odds of being in a higher BMI category when compared with the
children of authoritative fathers ( Wake, Nicholson, Hardy, & Smith, 2007 ).
Another study found that, compared with children of authoritative mothers,
children raised by authoritarian, permissive and neglectful mothers had a
significant increased odds of being overweight ( Rhee, et al. 2006 ). A survey
from Latino parents and their children suggested the association between children's
healthy eating & physical activity and parental use of positive reinforcement &
monitoring. It was also found out that appropriate disciplining styles application in
parents was associated with healthy diet, while parental use of control styles was
related to unhealthy diet ( Arredondo, et al. , 2006 ).

## 2. 5. 3    Chinese parenting style and childhood obesity

As the theories and models for parenting were developed based on the sample
of White Europeans and Americans, an important research question " is the

241

influence of parenting style different in different culture contexts?" was raised by several researchers. Chao believed that the concepts of authoritative and authoritarian were a little bit ethnocentric and do not capture the important characteristics of Chinese parenting style. He is also the first researcher to use the Chinese term "guan" which probably as "training", "to govern", "to care for" in a international parenting literature (Chao, 1994). In China, Confucianism was the most important part in traditional Chinese education during the past 2000 years. Although, during the past 3 decades, Chinese society has been greatly influenced by the culture from western countries, many Chinese's beliefs, behaviors and parenting style were still influenced by both Confucianism (Holroyd, 2003; P. Wu, et al., 2002; Xu, et al., 2005). Chinese parenting was often considered as "restrictive", "controlling" and "authoritarian" (Lin & Fu, 1990; Steinberg, et al., 1992). In fact, Confucian tradition accords family relationships with special significance. In a traditional Chinese family, sons or daughters should be loyal and respect to their parents (Bond & Hwang, 1986). Research indicated that, Americans value "nurturing innate ability", but Chinese attach importance to high self-discipline, obedience to parents, high parental involvement and sacrifice, which are deeply rooted in the Chinese traditional culture (Chao, 1994; F. M. Chen & Luster, 2002).

Chinese parenting style influenced by Confucianism was reported to be associated with children's social and school performance (X. Y. Chen, Dong, & Zhou, 1997; Nelson, et al., 2006) as well as child temperament (Porter, et al., 2005). However, only a few studies investigated the association between the Chinese parenting behaviors, parenting style and their children's weight status. For example, A cross-sectional study based on 163 Chinese children (aged 8 to 10 years) and their mothers indicated a positive relationship between democratic parenting and the children's BMI (J. L. Chen & Kennedy, 2004). Another study in Hong Kong found that parental influences, especially father's role modeling, could significantly influence overweight Chinese children's attraction to physical activity (Lau, et al., 2007).

On the other hand, the implementation of the single-child family planning program in the 1970s in mainland China may not only leaded to a great decrease in Chinese's natural growth rate of population ( Jing, 1994 ), but could also modify millions of Chinese's parenting behaviors and parenting styles. During the past 3 decades, as there is only one child in most Chinese family, many children could be spoiled by their parents and other family members. On the other hand, Chinese had also been exposed and influenced by western culture during the past 30 years. Therefore, Chinese parenting style rooted in traditional Chinese culture could be different now. In addition, in Chinese culture, mothers and fathers could play different roles and may have different parenting styles. Chinese mothers are always described as "Ci" ( kind ), while Chinese fathers are always regarded as "Yan" ( strict ) ( Berndt, et al. , 1993 ). However, little is known whether the influence of maternal parenting style and paternal parenting style on children's weight status is different and further studies are still needed to explore the relationship between Chinese parenting style and childhood obesity.

In general, during the past three decades, Chinese parenting style was influenced by traditional Chinese culture as well as the western culture. Although the differences between parenting styles in China and United States were reported, the theory of Chinese parenting style is still not well established. In addition, the theory of parenting established based on American parents ( Baumrind, 1971 ) was still widely applied in the studies on Chinese parents' parenting ( X. Y. Chen, et al. , 1997; Pong, Johnston, & Chen, 2009; Porter, et al. , 2005 ), which indicated that the theory still could be used to solve many research problems in Chinese parents.

## 2. 6　Home environment

### 2. 6. 1　Food availability and accessibility

Parents may also influence children's weight by changing home environment. An animal experimental study showed that the rats provided with five bottles of food and one bottle of water became fatter than the rats given five bottles of water and one of food, which indicated that the changes in food availability rather than physiological mechanisms maybe responsible for the unhealthy food intake and weight problem (Tordoff, 2002). Therefore, it also suggested that the issue of food availability at home should be included in childhood obesity interventions.

Recent studies indicated that food availability and accessibility as one of the most important determinants for fruit and vegetables consumption in children (Blanchette & Brug, 2005). For example, several cross sectional studies had shown that home availability of fruits and vegetables could predict fruit and vegetable consumption in school aged children and adolescents (Cullen, et al., 2003; Neumark-Sztainer, Wall, Perry, & Story, 2003). On the other hand, lack of nutritionally adequate and safe foods may increase risk for obesity and health problems (Adams, Grummer-Strawn, & Chavez, 2003). Another longitudinal study also suggested that home availability of fruits and vegetables is a very important predictor of fruit and vegetable intake (Larson, et al., 2007). In addition, not only food availability but also food accessibility is important for children's food consumption. For instance, it was found out that children were more likely to eat carrots if they were cut up into small pieces and placed in the place within children's reach (Hearn, et al., 1998). Therefore, to promote children's healthy food consumption, parents are advised to make healthy foods available and accessible at home.

As it had proved that fast food availability may contribute to increase in obesity prevalence (Jeffery & French, 1998), besides providing access to healthy foods, parents may also need to control their children's unhealthy foods intake through limiting the availability of such foods at home. Although it was reported that restricting access may arouse children's attention on restricted foods, and increase children's desire to eat those foods (Fisher & Birch, 1999b), most successful behavioral intervention programs to weight loss still include stimulus control techniques that involve limiting the availability of unhealthy foods at home (Young, Northern, Lister, Drummond, & O'Brien, 2007). Therefore, in spite of the negative effects, unhealthy food control is still suggested for the parents of obese or overweight children (Hughes, et al., 2008).

## 2. 6. 2　Home and neighborhood environment for physical activity

### 2. 6. 2. 1　Exercise equipment accessibility

Parents could promote children's physical activity in various ways. Research showed that adolescents' exercise equipment availability at home were positively associated with their physical activity level ( Dunton, Jamner, & Cooper, 2003 ). It was also found that physical activity participation among adolescent girls could be promoted by their perception of equipment that is accessible at home ( Motl, Dishman, Saunders, Dowda, & Pate, 2007 ). However, the data of another study showed that girls' access to sporting equipment at home is not significantly correlated to objectively measured moderate intensity physical activity ( Trost, Pate, Ward, Saunders, & Riner, 1999 ). It was also reported that equipment accessibility showed a statistically significant cross-sectional, but not longitudinal and direct influence on physical activity ( Motl, et al. , 2005 ). In general, although exercise equipment accessibility may not be a major determinant for childhood obesity prevention, it was suggested that the exercise equipment accessibility should be considered in the development of interventions for childhood obesity control.

### 2. 6. 2. 2　Home and neighborhood environment for physical activity

Research on the influence of the physical environment on obesity suggested that residents from communities with higher density, greater connectivity, and more land use mix were more likely to be physical active ( walking/cycling ) than the residents in low-density, poorly connected, and single land communities ( Saelens, Sallis, Black, & Chen, 2003 ). In addition, proximity to play space or recreational facilities, sidewalk availability, fast-food proximity and number of fast food stores et al. had also been thought to the determinants of the development of obesity ( Papas, et al. , 2007 ). However, most of these studies were based on adults. In the recent 10 years, the effects of built environment on childhood obesity also received some attention. For instance, playgrounds were reported to promote children's moderate to vigorous physical activity especially for girls ( Zask, van Beurden, Barnett, Brooks, & Dietrich, 2001 ). It was also found that residents of low walkability neighborhoods had higher BMI and were more likely to have overweight problems than the residents of high-walkability neighborhoods ( Saelens, et al. , 2003 ). In addition, research on Chinese showed that adolescents living in neighborhoods without sidewalks had significant higher odds to be physically inactive ( M. Li, Dibley, Sibbritt, & Yan, 2006 ). However, the data another study showed that overweight was not related to proximity to sports fields and fast food restaurants or the neighborhood crime level ( Burdette & Whitaker, 2004 ).

Neighborhood safety is another important factor that may influence parents' decision on children's physical activity. Many children complained that, because of the safety issue ( crossing busy roads etc. ), they were not allowed by parents to cycle or play out far from their home ( Mulvihill, et al. , 2000 ). One study had examined the determinants considered in parents' decisions about the selection of play spaces for their children ( Sallis, McKenzie, Elder, Broyles, & Nader, 1997 ). The results showed that safety is one of the most important factors that parents would consider. However, in a cross-sectional survey in 20 large US cities, mothers' perception of neighborhood safety was related to their children's screen time but not be associated with their children's time spent in outdoor play or risk for obesity ( Burdette & Whitaker, 2005 ). Another study also revealed that perceived neighborhood safety was not direct or indirect associated with self-reported physical activity ( Motl, et al. , 2007 ).

In general, although there were several studies indicated that physical environment maybe not significantly associated with physical activity, most research findings supported the importance of the home and neighborhood environments for children's physical activity promotion ( Franzini, et al. , 2009 ).

## 2. 7 Other related factors

### 2. 7. 1 Child's age and sensitive periods

As sensitive periods for development of childhood obesity may provide windows of opportunities prevention and treatment of obesity, it is very important to find the sensitive periods for influence of parents on childhood obesity. It was believed that the stage of cognitive development in children could be the most effective period for the behavior modification in childhood obesity prevention. Several potential critical or sensitive periods for development of childhood obesity was determined ( Dietz, 1994 ).

Mother's pregnancy could be one of the sensitive periods for intervention. It was found that infants exposed to acute malnutrition in early pregnancy are more likely to have overweight problem in later life ( Strauss, 1997 ). The research based on animal model also suggested that the control of energy utilization during early post-weaning period could be determined by the nutrient availability during the first 2 wk of intrauterine life ( Anguita, Sigulem, & Sawaya, 1993 ). In addition, maternal smoking during pregnancy might be a risk factor for childhood obesity ( Toschke, Montgomery, Pfeiffer, & von Kries, 2003; Von Kries, Toschke, Koletzko, & Slikker, 2002 ). Maternal diabetes during pregnancy was also found to be associated with childhood obesity ( Dabelea, et al. , 2008 ). Therefore, one of the key strategies for mother in childhood obesity prevention is to quit smoking and prevent diabetes during pregnancy. Although intrauterine factors may not make an important contribution to the children's BMI ( Smith, et al. , 2007 ), pregnancy still a sensitive period for the development of childhood obesity.

Infancy, when children are establishing the foundation for eating habits and nutritional adequacy for a life time ( Westenhoefer, 2002 ), is another sensitive period that parents need to pay attention to childhood obesity development. In this period, most research concentrated on whether breastfeeding is related to childhood obesity. For instance, it was indicated that breastfeeding may protect against obesity if maintained for 6 month ( Toschke, et al. , 2007 ). A cross-sectional study in German also found breastfeeding as a significant protective factor against the development of obesity ( Von Kries, et al. , 1999 ). One possible mechanism for protective effects of breastfeeding is that the breastfeeding helps infants learn how to regulate their energy intake than bottle-feeding does ( Lindsay, et al. , 2006 ). However, a longitudinal study based on 1958 "British Birth Cohort" ( n = 12, 857 ) found no relationship between breast feeding and

BMI in childhood ( Parsons, Power, & Manor, 2003 ). This study also showed that breastfeeding was protective against increased BMI in adults, but this influence disappear and no longer significant after confounding factors ( parental weight status, socioeconomic status etc. ) were controlled. In addition, a recent study did not support the association between breastfeeding promotion intervention and reduced childhood obesity as well ( Kramer, et al. , 2008 ). Although inconsistent results were found on the influence of breastfeeding on childhood obesity, it is still recommended that exclusive breastfeeding ( breast milk only, with no water, other fluids, or solids) for six months, with supplemental breast feeding continuing for at least two years ( Hoddinott, Tappin, & Wright, 2008 ).

Early childhood, when the physical activity and dietary patterns become more like adults' and dietary and physical activity habits are gradually established, could also be one of the important sensitive periods for the influence of parents on childhood obesity. Although the early learning is influenced by children's genetic predispositions ( Birch & Fisher, 1998 ), subsequent learning could be more important in the development of children's food choice ( Westenhoefer, 2002 ). Therefore, parents could play a key role in their children's learning process ( the influence of parents' belief, knowledge, behavior and parenting style on childhood obesity was reviewed above ). However, the influence of parents on childhood obesity may decrease when children grow up. For instance, it was reported that parental obesity significantly increased the risk of adult obesity among both obese and nonobese children under 10 years of age. But among older children, weight status in childhood becomes an increasingly important predictor of adult obesity, no matter the parents are obese or not ( Whitaker, et al. , 1997 ). Another study also suggested that obese 3 – 9 years olds children with obese parents may be ideal candidates for treatment, because the parents still have the chance to mold and shape their children's behaviors in their early childhood ( Epstein, et al. , 1990 ). However, after 10 years of age, parental influence has a significantly less influence on a child's risk of future weight problem.

## 2. 7. 2  Socioeconomic status

Family socioeconomic status (SES), which is normally determined by children's parents' income, education and occupations, could be another factor modifying the influence of parents on childhood obesity. It was also not hard to imagine that parents with low SES were less likely to buy fresh fruits and vegetable, exercise equipments & sports wear with good quality, and less likely to provide safe and high-walkability neighborhood for their children. In fact, it is widely accepted that, SES is one of the factors influencing childhood obesity, although the relationship between obesity and SES could be different in developed and developing countries  For instance, in the United States, it was reported that adolescents in the high SES group had lower odds to be obesity and overweight. In contrast, adolescents in low SES groups in China were found to have a lower odds to be obesity and overweight (Y. Wang, 2001). The present studies suggested that, in developed countries, low-SES groups are more likely to be obese than their high-SES counterparts, whereas low-SES groups have lower risk than high-SES groups in developing countries (McLaren, 2007; Y. Wang, 2001). In addition, the relation between SES and childhood obesity also differed by race/ethnicity (Whitaker & Orzol, 2006). Recent findings indicated that the reverse association (high-SES groups had low odds for overweight than are their low-SES counterparts) only existed in white children, not in black children and adolescents (Y. Wang & Zhang, 2006). However, most studies on SES were cross-sectional, and may not be able to demonstrate the long term relationship between SES and risks for obesity. Several longitudinal studies of SES and weight change over time were reported only among adults in developed societies (Ball & Crawford, 2005b). More longitudinal studies among children especially in developing countries were still needed. In general, it seems that childhood obesity may influenced by SES, but the relationship between SES and obesity varies across countries and ethnicity.

However, few of studies investigated the mechanisms that may explain the relations. The mechanisms by which SES are associated with obesity are still not clear. A number of potential mechanisms were suggested by several studies. For instance, the low prevalence of obesity in lower SES groups in developing societies was believed to be due to food insufficiency, perhaps together with high energy expenditure during manual work. In developing countries, a greater prevalence of obesity in individuals of higher SES could be due to their adequate food supplies, and maybe coupled with different cultural belief toward body shapes (Sobal & Stunkard, 1989). For developed countries, some researchers attempted to explain the effects of SES on obesity by investigating the role of behaviors. The summarized potential mediators may include low SES parents' poorer knowledge on physical activity and nutrition, poorer behavioral skills, differing social norms related to obesity and poorer access to healthy foods among lower SES areas et al. (Ball & Crawford, 2005b). For example, it was found significant differences in nutrition knowledge between socio-demographic groups, and knowledge was found to decline with lower educational level and socio-economic status (Parmenter, Waller, & Wardle, 2000). Another study showed that SES was inversely associated with calories intake; and positively related to weight concern as well as perceived social support for healthy diet and physical activity (Jeffery & French, 1996). A theoretical model was proposed to explain socio-cultural variations in food intake, exercise, and ultimately weight status (Ball & Crawford, 2005a). However, research also indicated that SES differences in these behaviors may not adequately explain SES differences in BMI (Ball, Mishra, & Crawford, 2003). It appears that additional studies are still needed to elucidate the possible mechanism for the association between SES and childhood obesity.

## 2. 8   Intervention

Many studies had demonstrated the importance of parents' involvement in weight loss programs, and therefore, parents' participation and support were highlighted in childhood obesity prevention (Barlow & the Expert Committee, 2007). Some experts even pointed out that if one or both parents are not involved in the intervention, the treatment is not likely to success (Dietz & Robinson, 2005).

School-based, family based, and community based intervention are the most common programs for childhood obesity. In many of studies, intervention through parents was only a part of a more comprehensive program ( Lindsay, et al. , 2006 ). Most of these multi-component interventions can be effective in childhood obesity treatment ( Foster, et al. , 2008 ; Robertson, et al. , 2008 ). A ten years longitudinal study showed that, the intervention in which children were treated together with their parents were more effective than the intervention only concentrated on children ( Epstein, et al. , 1990 ). A systematic review also indicated that the more behavior modification skills taught to both parents and children, the higher probability that the weight loss program is successful ( McLean, et al. , 2003 ). However, as these intervention programs were comprehensive programs mixed with various interventions targeted children, teachers, classmates, parents or other family members, it is impossible to figure out the effectiveness of intervention toward parents.

Recently, a special intervention integrating behavioral, social learning, and family system approaches toward childhood obesity was proposed, in which change was taken place in parents ( instead of the obese child ) addressing a healthy lifestyle rather than weight reduction ( Golan & Weizman, 2001 ). One of the advantages of this parents focused intervention is preventing the adverse psychological effects in conventional treatments. For instance, intervention toward obesity maybe sometimes not only related to food intake and physical activity but also associated with issues of shame and social isolation ( Sjoberg, Nilsson, & Leppert, 2005 ). While this problem could be avoided if parents focused program is applied.

On the other hand, the results application of these parents focused programs showed that this approach that targeted solely parents leaded to greater weight loss in obese children when compared with conventional intervention at treatment termination and at 1 - , 2 - , and 7 - year follow-up visits ( Golan & Crow, 2004b ). The feasibility of changing parental behaviors through multidimensional education in parents focused program had also been demonstrated ( McGarvey, et al. , 2004 ). In addition, some other studies using similar ideas resulted in great success as well. For instance, a recent study showed that overweight and obese mothers who modified their food choices and eating habits made comparable changes for their children (Klohe-Lehman, et al., 2007). Another study reported that obese child z-BMI change in a family based intervention program could be predicted by parent Z-BMI change (Wrotniak, et al., 2004).

However, there are still several limitations for the conceptual model for the parents focused intervention (Golan & Weizman, 2001). First of all, most interventions were focused on nutrition issues. Physical activity had not been valued as it should be. In addition, parents showed strong influences, mainly on the children no more than 12 years old. When children grow up, they become more independent, and their friends' influence becomes increasingly important (Golan & Weizman, 2001). Therefore, parents focused intervention provided a framework to guide future interventions and evaluations on childhood obesity, but improvements and adjustments are still needed.

## 2.9 Summary

The role of parents in the development and prevention of childhood obesity is multifaceted and complex. Current studies regarding the influence of parents on childhood obesity showed that parents played a critical role in the etiology of childhood obesity. Parents could influence children's weight status through the heredity, parents' perception, parenting behaviors, parenting styles, home environment et al. Given the considerable evidence for the association between parents and childhood obesity, it is suggested that influence of parents should receive more attention in childhood obesity intervention program.

# CHAPTER 3 EXAMINATION OF VALIDITY AND RELIABILITY OF QUESTIONNAIRES FOR CHINESE ADOLESCENTS AND PARENTS TO MEASURE PARENTS' PERCEPTION OF THEIR CHILDREN's WEIGHT, PARENTING BEHAVIORS AND PARENTING STYLE

## 3.1 Introduction

As childhood obesity was found to be one of the key predictors of adult obesity ( Whitaker, et al. , 1997 ) and could be associated with some chronic diseases ( Gunnell, et al. , 1998 ), children's weight problem has been regarded as an increasing important public health issue. Studies in the past two decades highlighted the importance of parents. It was found that parent may play a very important role in etiology, prevention and treatment of childhood obesity through their parenting behaviors and parenting styles ( Epstein, et al. , 1990; Lindsay, et al. , 2006 ).

Several studies had been done to investigate the association between parents' perception of their children's weight, parenting behaviors, parenting styles and childhood obesity in Chinese and some interesting results were found ( J. L. Chen & Kennedy, 2004; G. S. Ma, 2005; W. J. Ma, et al. , 2001 ). For example, it was reported that democratic parenting style, poor communication and poor behavior control could contribute to children's weight problem ( J. L. Chen & Kennedy, 2004 ). However, one of the limitations for the Chinese studies on this field is few valid and reliable questionnaires in Chinese were developed to measure Chinese parents' parenting behaviors and parenting style. Moreover, in many of these studies, only one or two parenting behaviors rather than a broader range of parenting behaviors were measured.

Although a number of valid and reliable questionnaire and scales, such as Child Feeding Questionnaire (CFQ), Family Eating and Activity Habits Questionnaire, and Caregiver's Feeding Styles Questionnaire, were well developed in western countries (Birch, et al., 2001; Golan & Weizman, 1998; Hughes, et al., 2003), these questionnaires could not be directly applied in Chinese population without reliability and validity test.

Therefore, the purpose of this study is to examine the validity and reliability of questionnaires to measure parenting behaviors, patents' perception of their children's weight and parenting styles for Chinese.

## 3. 2　Methods

### 3. 2. 1　Questionnaire selection

Relevant studies and questionnaire were reviewed to determine the theory framework as well as the advantages and shortcomings of the existing instruments (Golan & Weizman, 2001; Hughes, et al., 2008; Lindsay, et al., 2006; Rhee, 2008; Trost, et al., 2003). As there were dozens of possible questionnaires that could be applied to measure parents' perception of their children's weight, parenting behaviors and parenting styles, the questionnaires were selected based on the following 3 rules: 1) the questionnaire was proven to have at least acceptable validity and reliability; 2) the items are appropriate for adolescents aged 10 – 15; 3) there is no cultural conflict in the items.

*Adolescents' perception of weight*

Figure drawings incorporating boys, girls, men and women figures were applied to measure adolescents' perception of their and their parents' weight status (Collins, 1991). Each set of drawings consists of a set of seven figures, in which

254

the adolescent (or adult) is from very thin to very obese. Adolescents were asked to report their current body weight and the weight status they would like to be. The drawings were designed for children, but it could be applied in children over 10 years old as well (Parkinson, Tovée, & Cohen-Tovée, 1998). The test-retest reliability of this item based on Grade 1 – 3 children with 3 days internal was 0.71 (Collins, 1991).

### Parents' perception of their children's weights

To assess the parents' perceptions of their children's weights, an item applied in a previous study in China (Shi, Liena, Nirmal Kumara, & Holmboe-Ottesen, 2007) was selected in the current study. Parents were asked to report their children's weights subjectively by giving any one of the five possible answers: "very underweight", "slightly underweight", "normal", "slightly overweight", and "overweight".

### Parenting behaviors

Items applied to measure parent-reported parenting behaviors were modified based on the questionnaires used in previous studies (Arredondo, et al., 2006; O'Connor, et al., 2010), was used to assess the parenting behaviors. The scale had the following subscales: "Diet and physical activity (PA) Monitoring", "Use food or sedentary behaviors as rewards", "Pressure to eat", "Restricting access to unhealthy food and sedentary behaviors", and "Reinforcement" regarding adolescents' eating and PA. Five Likert-scale responses were provided for these questions (response options: never, rarely, sometimes, frequently, always or strongly disagree, disagree, neutral, agree, strongly agree).

### Perceived parenting style

As parenting style would provide the expected effects only when they are actually perceived by the adolescents (Choquet, Hassler, Morin, Falissard, & Chau, 2008), the items used to measure adolescents' perceived parenting styles in Authoritative Parenting Index (API) were used in the current study. The

Authoritative Parenting Index was reported to be had a factor structure consistent with a theoretical model of the construct and had good reliability (Jackson, Henriksen, & Foshee, 1998). API could be applied in fourth grade (9 – 10 years old) to tenth grade (15 – 16 years old) children (Jackson, et al. , 1998). There are nine items in the responsiveness subscale and seven items in the demandingness subscale.

### 3.2.2 Translation and Back-translation

The procedure of the translation and back translation, based on steps introduced in cross-cultural translation technique (Banville, Desrosiers, & Ganet-Volet, 2000) was performed for the items derived from questionnaire in English. The items were translated into simplified Chinese by two bilingual graduate students. Their two translation versions were compared after the translation is completed. Differences between the two versions were discussed, and finally reached an agreement. After that, another two bilingual graduate students back-translated the instrument into English, and neither of them was given the original version beforehand. The same strategy in translation was also applied in the back-translation. The back translations were compared to the original version to ensure the accuracy of translation for instruction, each item and response option.

### 3.2.3 Content validity

Based on the conceptual framework of parenting behaviors and parenting styles, a pool of items were prepared. Five experts in family studies, nutrition, sports science, physical education and medicine were invited to evaluate the content validity of questionnaire. The experts were informed about the objectives of the questionnaires. They were required to complete an evaluation form for the questionnaire on an individual basis. They rated the effectiveness of each item, add some important factors that were omitted in the questionnaire, and evaluated the feasibility of the questionnaire application in Chinese adolescents and parents. The items with less than 80% agreement (four out of five experts agreed to keep the item) were dropped. The questionnaire was modified according to the reviewers.

### 3.2.4　Pretest of the experimental version

15 pairs of adolescents and their parents at Ganzhou and Shantou (7 pairs in Ganzhou and 8 pairs in Shantou) were invited to complete the experimental version of questionnaire followed by a short interview. At first, according to the procedure recommended by Banville et al. (2000), the adolescents and parents were invited to complete the experimental version of questionnaire. They were invited to indicate the questionnaire words they do not understand or feel uncomfortable. They were also invited to talk about their (or their parents') parenting behaviors and styles, and whether the items catch their parenting behaviors and styles. According to their feedbacks, the content and language of some items were modified so as to make the questionnaire culturally relevant.

### 3.2.5　Test-retest reliability and internal consistency

As it was reported that reasonable precision for estimates of reliability needs at least 50 study participants (Hopkins, 2000), 127 pairs of adolescents and their parents (Ganzhou: 62 pairs, Shantou: 65 pairs) were recruited. During the reliability study, adolescents and their parents were required to complete the questionnaires twice with two weeks apart, so that the test-retest reliability, internal reliability could be determined.

### 3.2.6　Construct validity

2,162 pairs of adolescents and parents in Ganzhou and Shantou were invited to participate in a survey using the questionnaire. 1,000 data extracted randomly from the survey was analyzed for construct validity.

### 3.2.7　Data analysis

The test-retest reliability of each item was determined by intraclass correlation coefficient (ICC). ICC was regarded as acceptable if ICC was greater than 0.7. Cronbach's alpha was performed to determine internal reliability of the scaled responses to multiple items. Internal consistency was deemed acceptable if Cronbach's alpha is greater than 0.6 (Sim & Wright, 2000). Confirmatory Factor Analysis (CFA) using Lisrel 8.51 software was conducted to determine construct validity. Non-Normed Fit Index (NNFI) ( >0.90 indicates good fit),

Comparative Fit Index (CFI) ( >0.90 indicates good fit) and Root Mean Square Error of Approximation (RMSEA) ( <0.08 indicates acceptable fit) were used for determining model fit (Hooper, Coughlan, & Mullen, 2008).

## 3.3 Results

### 3.3.1 Content validity

A total of 46 items and 41 items were proposed for questionnaire for adolescents and their parent respectively. 6 items in adolescent questionnaire and 3 items in parent questionnaire, which were lower than 80% agreement in content validity test, were dropped. Therefore, after content validity test, 40 items and 38 items were retained for questionnaire for adolescents and their parent respectively.

### 3.3.2 Test-retest reliability and internal consistency

The demographic information of the participants in the reliability test were summarized in the Table 3.1. Of the 127 adolescents, 65 (51.2%) were boys and 60 (48.8%) were girls. The age of the adolescents ranged from 10 to 15 years old. 80 out of the 127 parents (63%) recruited in the reliability study were mothers.

**Table 3.1　Demographic data ( N = 127 )**

| | |
|---|---|
| Child sex, % | |
| 　Boy | 51.2 |
| 　Girl | 48.8 |
| Child age, mean ±SD, y | 13.1 ±0.8 |
| Height, cm | 162.2 ±6.7 |
| Weight, kg | 50.2 ±7.6 |
| BMI | 19.1 ±2.4 |
| Overweight, % | 18.1 |
| Parent sex, % | |
| 　Male | 37.0 |
| 　Female | 63.0 |

As it was showed in the Table 3. 2, the two weeks test-retest reliability of the items on adolescents' and parents' perception of adolescents' weight were excellent, which ranged from 0. 83 to 0. 92. The results indicated that the items on adolescents' and parents' perception of adolescents' weight status were reliable.

**Table 3. 2  The test retest reliability of the items related to adolescents' and their parents' perception of adolescents' weight status**

| Items | ICC | 95% CI | N | P | Report Status |
|---|---|---|---|---|---|
| Which picture looks the most like how you look? | 0. 92 | 0. 89 – 0. 95 | 123 | . 000 | A |
| Which picture looks the most like the way you want to look? | 0. 86 | 0. 80 – 0. 90 | 123 | . 000 | A |
| Which picture looks the most like your father? | 0. 91 | 0. 87 – 0. 94 | 123 | . 000 | A |
| Which picture looks the most like your mother? | 0. 91 | 0. 87 – 0. 94 | 123 | . 000 | A |
| Which picture looks shows the way you want to look when you grow up. | 0. 83 | 0. 76 – 0. 88 | 123 | . 000 | A |
| Please report the weight status of your child | 0. 88 | 0. 82 – 0. 92 | 126 | . 000 | P |

Note: A: adolescent-reported; P: parent-reported

For the test-retest reliability of items on parenting behaviors, only one item was found to be less than 0. 7 and was dropped (Table 3. 3). The results showed that the test-retest reliability of other items ranged from 0. 71 to 0. 83, and the internal consistencies of subscales ranged from 0. 69 to 0. 79. The results suggested that the questionnaire was reliable and internal consistent.

**Table 3. 3  The test retest reliability and internal consistency of the items on parenting behaviors**

| Items | ICC | 95% CI | N | P | Cronbach's α |
|---|---|---|---|---|---|
| **Diet and physical activity (PA) monitoring** | | | | | 0. 76 |
| 1. How much do you keep track of sweets (candy, ice cream, cake) that your child eats? | 0. 74 | 0. 61 – 0. 82 | 125 | . 000 | |
| 2. How much do you keep track of the high-fat foods that your child eats? | 0. 71 | 0. 57 – 0. 80 | 125 | . 000 | |

| Items | ICC | 95% CI | N | P | Cronbach's α |
|---|---|---|---|---|---|
| 3. How much do you keep track of servings of fruits and vegetables your child is eating? | 0.80 | 0.70 – 0.86 | 125 | .000 | |
| 4. How often must your child ask permission before getting a snack? | 0.71 | 0.56 – 0.80 | 125 | .000 | |
| 5. How much do you keep track of the amount of TV or videos your child is watching? | 0.72 | 0.59 – 0.81 | 125 | .000 | |
| 6. How much do you keep track of exercise your child is getting? | 0.73 | 0.60 – 0.81 | 125 | .000 | |
| **Reinforcement** | | | | | 0.79 |
| 7. How often do you praise your child for eating a healthy snack? | 0.83 | 0.75 – 0.89 | 123 | .000 | |
| 8. How often do you praise your child for being physically active? | 0.71 | 0.57 – 0.81 | 122 | .000 | |
| **Use food or sedentary behaviors as rewards** | | | | | 0.69 |
| 9. I offer sweets (candy, ice cream, cake) to my child as a reward for good behavior | 0.77 | 0.66 – 0.84 | 125 | .000 | |
| 10. I offer TV, or video game to my child as a reward for good behavior | 0.72 | 0.60 – 0.81 | 125 | .000 | |
| **Pressure to eat** | | | | | 0.74 |
| 11. My child should always eat all the food on his/her plate | 0.55 | 0.34 – 0.70 | 126 | .000 | D |
| 12. I have to be especially careful to make sure my child eats enough | 0.76 | 0.65 – 0.84 | 126 | .000 | |
| 13. If my child says "I am not hungry" I try to get him/her to eat anyway | 0.78 | 0.67 – 0.85 | 124 | .000 | |
| 14. If I don't regulate or guide my child's eating, he/she would eat much less than he/she should | 0.71 | 0.56 – 0.80 | 124 | .000 | |
| **Restricting access to unhealthy food and sedentary behaviors** | | | | | 0.74 |
| 15. I limit the amount of soda my child drinks | 0.71 | 0.57 – 0.81 | 124 | .000 | |
| 16. I limit the number of snacks my child eats | 0.71 | 0.57 – 0.80 | 124 | .000 | |
| 17. I limit the amount of time my child watches TV or videos during week (Mon-Fri) | 0.81 | 0.73 – 0.87 | 124 | .000 | |
| 18. I limit the amount of time my child watches TV or videos during weekend (Sat/Sun) | 0.83 | 0.75 – 0.89 | 124 | .000 | |

Note: D: The item was deleted, Cronbach's α was calculated based on the items with test-retest reliability higher than 0.70

The results of test-retest reliability and internal consistencies in the items of parenting style were also found to be acceptable. As it was showed in Table 3.4 and Table 3.5, the test-retest reliability of 16 items ranged from 0.70 to 0.84 for mothers and 0.70 to 0.85 for fathers. The internal consistencies of responsiveness and demandingness for parents ranged from 0.70 to 0.75, demonstrating that the questionnaire was reliable and internal consistent.

**Table 3.4   The test retest reliability and internal consistency of
the items on adolescent-reported fathers' parenting style**

| Items | ICC | 95% CI | N | P | Cronbach's α |
|---|---|---|---|---|---|
| **Responsiveness (fathers)** | | | | | 0.70 |
| 1. He is always telling me what to do | 0.72 | 0.60 – 0.80 | 123 | .000 | |
| 2. He makes rules without asking what I think. | 0.75 | 0.64 – 0.82 | 123 | .000 | |
| 3. He makes me feel better when I am upset. | 0.71 | 0.59 – 0.80 | 123 | .000 | |
| 4. He is too busy to talk to me. | 0.75 | 0.64 – 0.82 | 123 | .000 | |
| 5. He listens to what I have to say. | 0.73 | 0.62 – 0.81 | 123 | .000 | |
| 6. He likes me just the way I am. | 0.71 | 0.57 – 0.79 | 123 | .000 | |
| 7. He tells me when I do a good job on things. | 0.78 | 0.69 – 0.85 | 123 | .000 | |
| 8. He wants to hear about my problems. | 0.76 | 0.65 – 0.83 | 123 | .000 | |
| 9. He is pleased with how I behave. | 0.82 | 0.74 – 0.87 | 123 | .000 | |
| **Demandingness (fathers)** | | | | | 0.75 |
| 10. He has rules that I must follow. | 0.72 | 0.60 – 0.81 | 123 | .000 | |
| 11. He tells me times when I must come home. | 0.72 | 0.60 – 0.81 | 123 | .000 | |
| 12. He makes sure I tell her where I am going. | 0.71 | 0.59 – 0.80 | 123 | .000 | |
| 13. He makes sure I go to bed on time. | 0.75 | 0.64 – 0.82 | 123 | .000 | |
| 14. He asks me what I do with friends. | 0.70 | 0.57 – 0.79 | 123 | .000 | |
| 15. He knows where I am after school. | 0.85 | 0.78 – 0.89 | 123 | .000 | |
| 16. He checks to see if I do my homework. | 0.75 | 0.64 – 0.83 | 123 | .000 | |

Note: D: The item was deleted, Cronbach's α was calculated based on the items with test-retest reliability higher than 0.70

Table 3.5  The test retest reliability and internal consistency of
the items on adolescent-reported mothers' parenting style

| Items | ICC | 95% CI | N | P | Cronbach's α |
|---|---|---|---|---|---|
| **Responsiveness (mothers)** | | | | | 0.71 |
| 1. She is always telling me what to do | 0.74 | 0.62 – 0.82 | 122 | .000 | |
| 2. She makes rules without asking what I think. | 0.75 | 0.65 – 0.83 | 123 | .000 | |
| 3. She makes me feel better when I am upset. | 0.72 | 0.59 – 0.80 | 123 | .000 | |
| 4. She is too busy to talk to me. | 0.70 | 0.58 – 0.79 | 123 | .000 | |
| 5. She listens to what I have to say. | 0.73 | 0.61 – 0.81 | 123 | .000 | |
| 6. She likes me just the way I am. | 0.70 | 0.57 – 0.79 | 123 | .000 | |
| 7. She tells me when I do a good job on things. | 0.84 | 0.76 – 0.89 | 123 | .000 | |
| 8. She wants to hear about my problems. | 0.76 | 0.65 – 0.83 | 123 | .000 | |
| 9. She is pleased with how I behave. | 0.73 | 0.61 – 0.81 | 122 | .000 | |
| **Demandingness (mothers)** | | | | | 0.71 |
| 10. She has rules that I must follow. | 0.74 | 0.63 – 0.82 | 123 | .000 | |
| 11. She tells me times when I must come home. | 0.70 | 0.56 – 0.79 | 123 | .000 | |
| 12. She makes sure I tell her where I am going. | 0.74 | 0.63 – 0.82 | 123 | .000 | |
| 13. She makes sure I go to bed on time. | 0.72 | 0.59 – 0.80 | 123 | .000 | |
| 14. She asks me what I do with friends. | 0.75 | 0.64 – 0.82 | 123 | .000 | |
| 15. She knows where I am after school. | 0.74 | 0.62 – 0.82 | 123 | .000 | |
| 16. She checks to see if I do my homework. | 0.70 | 0.58 – 0.79 | 123 | .000 | |

Note: D: The item was deleted, Cronbach's α was calculated based on the items with test-retest reliability higher than 0.70

After the reliability test, one item in parents' questionnaire was dropped, and a total of 40 items and 38 items were left in the questionnaires for adolescents and parents respectively.

### 3.3.3  Construct validity

As it was showed in Table 3.6, the results of CFA showed that the factor loadings of the items on parenting behaviors ranged from 0.60 to 0.76. The model exhibited acceptable fit indicated by the goodness-of-fit statistics ( RMSEA = 0. 052, NNFI = 0. 91, CFI = 0. 92). The results of CFA on parenting style items were summarized in Table 3. 7. The factors loading estimated based on the data of fathers and mothers were quite similar (ranged from 0. 55 to 0. 76 for fathers and ranged from 0. 59 to 0. 74 for mothers). The RMSEA, CFI and NNFI for the parenting style model also indicated acceptable fit.

### Table 3. 6 Factor loadings of confirmatory factor analysis on parenting behaviors items

| Items | Factor loading[a] |
|---|---|
| **Diet and physical activity ( PA ) monitoring** | |
| 1. How much do you keep track of sweets ( candy, ice cream, cake) that your child eats? | 0. 67 |
| 2. How much do you keep track of the high-fat foods that your child eats? | 0. 68 |
| 3. How much do you keep track of servings of fruits and vegetables your child is eating? | 0. 66 |
| 4. How often must your child ask permission before getting a snack? | 0. 72 |
| 5. How much do you keep track of the amount of TV or videos your child is watching? | 0. 69 |
| 6. How much do you keep track of exercise your child is getting? | 0. 74 |
| **Reinforcement** | |
| 7. How often do you praise your child for eating a healthy snack? | 0. 65 |
| 8. How often do you praise your child for being physically active? | 0. 70 |
| **Use food or sedentary behaviors as rewards** | |
| 9. I offer sweets ( candy, ice cream, cake) to my child as a reward for good behavior | 0. 76 |
| 10. I offer TV, or video game to my child as a reward for good behavior | 0. 65 |
| **Pressure to eat** | |
| 11. I have to be especially careful to make sure my child eats enough | 0. 71 |
| 12. If my child says "I am not hungry" I try to get him/her to eat anyway | 0. 70 |
| 13. If I don't regulate or guide my child's eating, he/she would eat much less than he/she would eat much less than he/she should | 0. 68 |

| Items | Factor loading[a] |
|---|---|
| **Restricting access to unhealthy food and sedentary behaviors** | |
| 14. I limit the amount of soda my child drinks | 0.60 |
| 15. I limit the number of snacks my child eats | 0.74 |
| 16. I limit the amount of time my child watches TV or videos during week (Mon-Fri) | 0.74 |
| 17. I limit the amount of time my child watches TV or videos during weekend (Sat/Sun) | 0.71 |

[a] The goodness-of-fit statistics of CFA: RMSEA = 0.052, NNFI = 0.91, CFI = 0.92

**Table 3.7  Factor loadings of confirmatory factor analysis on parenting style items**

| Item | Factor loading | |
|---|---|---|
| | Father | Mother |
| **Responsiveness** | | |
| 1. He/She is always telling me what to do | 0.64 | 0.65 |
| 2. He/She makes rules without asking what I think. | 0.64 | 0.66 |
| 3. He/She makes me feel better when I am upset. | 0.69 | 0.67 |
| 4. He/She is too busy to talk to me. | 0.62 | 0.61 |
| 5. He/She listens to what I have to say. | 0.68 | 0.66 |
| 6. He/She likes me just the way I am. | 0.65 | 0.69 |
| 7. He/She tells me when I do a good job on things. | 0.62 | 0.61 |
| 8. He/She wants to hear about my problems. | 0.55 | 0.59 |
| 9. He/She is pleased with how I behave. | 0.63 | 0.63 |
| **Demandingness** | | |
| 10. He/She has rules that I must follow. | 0.70 | 0.69 |
| 11. He/She tells me times when I must come home. | 0.62 | 0.66 |
| 12. He/She makes sure I tell her where I am going. | 0.72 | 0.73 |
| 13. He/She makes sure I go to bed on time. | 0.66 | 0.64 |
| 14. He/She asks me what I do with friends. | 0.76 | 0.74 |
| 15. He/She knows where I am after school. | 0.68 | 0.68 |
| 16. He/She checks to see if I do my homework. | 0.65 | 0.67 |

The goodness-of-fit statistics of CFA: RMSEA = 0.056, NNFI = 0.92, CFI = 0.93 (based on fathers); RMSEA = 0.055, NNFI = 0.93, CFI = 0.94 (based on mothers)

## 3.4 Discussion and conclusion

The purpose of this study is to determine the validity and reliability of the questionnaires for Chinese adolescents and parents to measure parents' perception of their children's weight status, parenting behaviors and parenting styles. The content validity, construct validity, 2 weeks test retest reliability and internal consistency of the questionnaires were determined in the present study. The results of the data indicated that the validity and reliability instruments were acceptable and could be applied in Chinese adolescents and their parents.

Some parents related behaviors, which could be associated with childhood obesity, were identified based on previous studies. For instance, recent studies emphasized the influences of parental feeding behaviors on the child's and infant's food intakes ( Koletzko, et al. , 2009; Kroller & Warschburger, 2009 ). Based on conceptual framework and the questionnaires used in previous studies ( Arredondo, et al. , 2006; O'Connor, et al. , 2010 ), the 17 items questionnaire was developed to measure parenting behaviors in Chinese parents. "Diet and PA monitoring", "reinforcement", "use food as rewards", "pressure to eat" and "restricting access to unhealthy food and sedentary behaviors", which were found to be the important parenting behaviors contributed to the development of childhood obesity ( Clark, et al. , 2007; Faith, Scanlon, et al. , 2004; Rhee, 2008 ), were included as the factors in this parenting behavior questionnaire. The goodness-of-fit statistics of CFA indicated that the model provided acceptable fit to the data in the current study. Moreover, content validity, two weeks test retest reliability and internal consistency were also found to be acceptable.

In the current study, the items for parenting style measurement, were developed based on Authoritative Parenting Index ( API ). Evidences were provided in support of the validity and reliability of the API ( Jackson, et al. , 1998 ). The results of CFA indicated that the structure of the questionnaire was consistent with the theory model of parenting style, in which parenting styles were conceptualized based on two underlying dimensions: demandingness and responsiveness (Baumrind, 1971). The results of content validity test and reliability test also proved that the questionnaire was valid in content and reliable. However, the cultural difference between China and western countries should be considered for parenting style. For instance, it was reported that Americans and Europeans attached importance to "nurturing innate ability". However, Chinese emphasized the importance of high self-discipline, obedience to parents, high parental involvement and sacrifice, which are rooted the Confucian education philosophy (Chao, 1994; F. M. Chen & Luster, 2002). Therefore, a Chinese researcher pointed out that the concepts of authoritative and authoritarian may not capture the important characteristics of Chinese parenting styles (Chao, 1994). In addition, there is no standard cutoff point for the questionnaires to measure parenting style, the four parenting styles were categorized based on a relative criterion rather than an absolute one, in which a cross-classification of high and low scores based on median splits on the responsiveness and demandingness subscale identified the four categorical parenting styles (Darling & Steinberg, 1993). This means that considering the difference in parenting style of Chinese and American parents (P. Wu, et al. , 2002), a neglectful mother in a Chinese study could be regarded as an authoritative mother if her data were included in a study in the United States. Additional studies were needed for the measurement of parenting style.

Several limitations in this study should be acknowledged when interpreted the data. First of all, as no specific theory on Chinese parenting was well established and could be applied in the present study, the questionnaires were still based on the theory established in western countries, although several steps were applied in the current study to make the questionnaire culturally relevant. Therefore, the questionnaire may not catch all the characteristics of Chinese parenting behaviors and parenting styles. Nevertheless, the theory of parenting established based on American parents (Baumrind, 1971) was still widely applied in the studies on Chinese parents' parenting (X. Y. Chen, et al. , 1997; Pong, et al. , 2009; Porter, et al. , 2005), which indicated that the theory still could be used to solve many research problems in Chinese parents. The questionnaires were still meaningful for the studies on the Chinese parenting. Secondly, memory problem is very hard to avoid in the test retest situations, although there was two weeks' time between the two reliability tests. The adolescents and parents may still remember some of their choices in the first test, and reproduce answers in the second test, which may lead to overestimation of the test retest reliability. Thirdly, although the parent, who was invited to complete the questionnaire in the second reliability test, was required to be the same parent in the first reliability test, it was still possible that several participants may not comply with the rules. In this case the test retest reliability could be underestimated. In addition, the participants recruited in this study were 10 – 15 years old adolescents and their parents in Ganzhou and Shantou. Therefore, the questionnaires developed in the current study may not be appropriate to be used in the children under ten years old or in other areas of China.

Evidences were provided in the current study for the content validity, construct validity, test retest reliability and internal consistency. Despite of the limitations of the study, it was still demonstrated that the questionnaires for both adolescents and parents were valid, reliable and could be applied in Chinese adolescents and their parents in southern China to measure parents' perception of their children's weight status, parenting behaviors and parenting styles.

# CHAPTER 4    PARENTING BEHAVIORS AND ADOLESCENT OBESITY

## 4. 1    Introduction

Although malnutrition among children remained prevalent in developing countries, it was reported that prevalence of overweight in young women is higher than the prevalence of underweight in many developing countries, especially in the countries with high economic growth ( Mendez, Monteiro, & Popkin, 2005 ). Recent research showed that Chinese children is experiencing large increase in mean BMI at the $95^{th}$ percentile ( Popkin, 2010 ), which indicated that, just like the trend in the United States, the childhood obesity is becoming an increasing important problem in China.

Balanced diet, increased physical activity and social support to alter modern diets and lifestyles were suggested to solve obesity epidemic ( Heber, 2010 ). The importance of parents' participation in weight control programs were also highlighted ( Barlow & the Expert Committee, 2007 ). It was suggested that treatments should be a family based program with the participation of at least one parent ( Dietz & Robinson, 2005; Robinson, 1999 ). Recent evidences in both qualitative and quantitative studies also confirmed the importance of parent involvement in the childhood obesity treatment ( Heinberg, et al. , 2009; Stewart, et al. , 2008 ).

Parents not only influence their children's diet and physical activity through the food & home environment they provide, their feeding behaviors ( restriction assess to some food, pressure to eat, using food as rewards etc. ), financial and emotional support for their children's sports participation, but also influence the development of children's dietary and exercise habits through role modeling. For instance, a longitudinal study demonstrated that parental restriction of food intake at age five could predict higher BMI at age seven, after BMI at age three was adjusted for ( Faith, Berkowitz, et al. , 2004 ). It could be explained that the children's attention and appetite for restricted foods was increased by their parents' restricting feeding strategies ( Fisher & Birch, 1999b ). The data from Framingham Children's Study showed that children of physically active parents had significantly higher odds to be to be physically active than the children of physically inactive mothers ( Moore, et al. , 1991 ).

However, inconsistent results were still found in several studies. For example, a study showed that adolescents who received parental reinforcement participated in significantly more days of physical activity in a week than did their counterparts who did not ( King, et al. , 2008 ). However, the data of another study showed that girl's perception of parent's support for physical activity was not associated with girl's activity levels ( Adkins, et al. , 2004 ). Therefore, further studies were still needed to clarify the parenting behaviors that associated with children's diet and physical activity, which could be very important in the prevention and treatment of childhood obesity.

The association between Chinese parenting behaviors and childhood obesity were also reported by some Chinese studies. For instance, a cross sectional study based on 930 families with 2 – to 6 – year – old children in Beijing revealed a strong association between parents' and children's dietary habits, TV watching and physical activity ( Jiang, et al. , 2006 ). Another study from 104 parents of overweight children in Hong Kong had showed that parental influence, especially father's role modeling, significantly influenced overweight Chinese children's physical activity participation ( Lau, et al. , 2007 ). However, most of these studies concentrated on one or two parenting behaviors rather than a broad range of parenting behaviors. In addition, the difference in cultural orientation toward parenting behaviors should be acknowledged. For example, in Chinese culture, Chinese mothers are always described as " Ci" ( kind), while Chinese fathers are always regarded as "Yan" (strict) (Berndt, et al. , 1993). Therefore, mothers and fathers could play different roles in family and may have different parenting behaviors. However, few studies in China compared diet and physical activity related parenting behaviors in fathers and mothers.

Therefore, the purposes of this study are 1) to determine the association between adolescents' dietary habits, physical activity, weight status and parenting behaviors; 2) to compared diet and physical activity related parenting behaviors in Chinese fathers and mothers.

## 4. 2    Methods

### Study population and procedure

The study population of present study was the adolescents and their parents in urban areas (city or town) of southern China, due to much higher prevalence of obesity in the urban areas as compared with rural areas (countryside) (Luo & Hu, 2002). As improved economic and social conditions was found to be an important factor that may lead to Chinese's increased nutrient-dense and energy-dense food intake, sedentary lifestyle and weight status (Y. Wang, Monteiro, & Popkin, 2002), it was decided to recruited our participants from a developed city and an underdeveloped city in southern China. Stratified random sampling was applied in the present study, in which a city (Shantou) in developed area and a city (Ganzhou) in underdeveloped area were chosen. Shantou, one of the original Special Economic Zones of China established in the 1980s, is one of the developed regions in southern China. The Gross Domestic Product (GDP) per capita in Shantou was 20,279 RMB (Shantou municipal bureau of statistics, 2010). Ganzhou, one of the old revolutionary base areas in China, is an underdeveloped inland city located in southern China. The GDP per capita in Ganzhou was 9,391 RMB (Ganzhou municipal bureau of statistics, 2010). Adolescents and their parents were randomly recruited from grade 1 and grade 2 of secondary schools in Ganzhou and Shantou respectively. For example, in Ganzhou, there are two districts. In the present study, a key secondary school and an ordinary secondary school was randomly chosen in each district. 4 - 6 classes in each school (2 - 3 classes in each grade) were randomly drawn in the investigation. The same sampling strategy was applied in Shantou. Exclusion criteria for adolescents were using medications that may influence weight gain or loss, and a diagnosis of physical or developmental disability or chronic illness.

From April to May 2009, 2,162 pairs of adolescents and parents participated in the present survey (Ganzhou: 1,179 pairs; Shantou: 1,106 pairs). There were 19 adolescents who had physical disability or received medications that influence their weight status were excluded from the analysis. 274 parents did not send the questionnaire back. Consequently, 2,143 adolescents and 1,869 their parents were finally included in the data analysis.

During the survey, adolescents in secondary school were invited to complete an anthropometric test for body weight and height, and were asked to fill out questionnaires inside a classroom with the assistance of investigators. The adolescents were also asked to take home the "questionnaires for parents" for either their mother or father to fill out, and to give the questionnaires back to our survey conductors. Souvenirs were given to the participants as compliments.

Other than the participants in the main survey, 127 pairs adolescents and parents (Ganzhou: 62 pairs, Shantou: 65 pairs) were invited to participate in a reliability study four weeks prior to the main survey. During the reliability study, adolescents and their parents were required to complete the questionnaires twice with two weeks apart. The test-retest reliability of each item and internal consistency was determined by intraclass correlation coefficient (ICC) and Cronbach's alpha respectively.

Signed informed consent was obtained from all participants (including adolescents and parents) prior to the survey. The adolescents and their parents were briefly introduced that they need to provide some information about their children's health status and were highly encouraged to honestly report what they really think and what they did. In the instruction of the questionnaire, both adolescents and parents were clearly informed that there is no right or wrong answers for each item and the questionnaire is anonymous. Formal approval was granted from the Chinese University of Hong Kong Research Ethics Committee.

## Main study measures

### Adolescent weight status

An adolescent's body weight to the nearest 0.1 kg was measured with minimal clothing and without shoes using a measuring scale. An adolescent's body height to the nearest 0.5 cm was taken using a stadiometer. An adolescent's body mass index (BMI) was calculated as his or her weight in kilograms divided by the square of his height in meters. The BMI was further categorized either as underweight (thinness, BMI-for-age < - 2 SD), normal, or overweight (BMI-for-age > 1SD) based on the international growth standards for school-aged children and adolescents updated by the World Health Organization (WHO) (Butte, et al., 2007; De Onis, et al., 2007). The age and gender specific BMI Z scores (Z-BMI) for each adolescent was calculated based on the international growth standard.

### Parent weight status

The BMIs of parents were recorded based on their self-reported heights and weights, as it is not feasible to measure parents' height and weight in the present study. Validity of self-reported heights and weights of adults were well reported (Bolton-Smith, Woodward, Tunstall-Pedoe, & Morrison, 2000; Wada, et al., 2005). Pearson's ratio between self-reported BMI and measured BMI was 0.943 and 0.950 for men and women, respectively (Wada, et al., 2005). According to the BMI reference for screening overweight and obesity among Chinese adults, parental BMIs were categorized either as non-overweight (BMI < 24kg/m$^2$) or overweight (24 kg/m$^2$ ≤ BMI < 28 kg/m$^2$), or obese (BMI ≥ 28 kg/m$^2$) (Zhou & Cooperative Meta-Analysis Group of the Working Group on Obesity in China, 2002).

### Adolescents' dietary habits

Adolescents' dietary habits were measured by a five-point Likert-scale including 12 items. During the survey, the adolescents were provided with responses ranging from "never," "rarely," "sometimes," "frequently," and "always" to indicate the frequency of their dietary behaviors during the past years. The sample questions were as follows: "I eat at least 3 servings of vegetables a day" and "I eat more during dinner if the food tastes good. " The total score of the adolescents' dietary habits was calculated as the sum score of each item ( several item were reversed coded). The validity and reliability of the scale were found to be acceptable ( Sheu, 2003 ). The reliability test in the current study showed that the two weeks test-retest reliability of these items ranged from 0. 70 to 0. 79. The internal consistency for this scale was 0. 71.

### Adolescents' physical activity level

All adolescents were invited to complete a validated physical activity rating questionnaire for children and youth ( PARCY ) to assess their average weekly physical activity over the last year. The PARCY is a 1-item activity rating modified from the Jackson Activity Coding ( Baumgartner & Jackson, 1996; George, Stone, & Burkett, 1997) and the Godin-Shephard Activity Questionnaire modified for Adolescents ( Aaron, et al. , 1993; Godin & Shephard, 1985 ). The criterion validity and convergent validity of PARCY have been published in other sources ( Hui, 2001; Hui, Chan, Wong, Ha, & Hong, 2001; Kong, et al. , 2010). The scale is an 11 − point scale ( 0 − 10) ranging from no exercise at all ( rating of 0) to vigorous exercise almost everyday ( rating of 10). The design of the rating took into consideration activity frequency, duration, and intensity. The physical activity levels of the subjects were further categorized into either "inactive" ( PARCY = 0 to 2 ), "slightly active" ( PARCY = 3 to 6 ), or "active" ( PARCY = 7 to 10) groups for analysis. The reliability test in the current study showed that the two weeks test-retest reliability of the item was 0. 83.

### Parent-reported parenting behaviors

An 17 − item, five-point Likert-type scale, which was modified and translated based on the questionnaires used in previous studies ( Arredondo, et al. , 2006; O'Connor, et al. , 2010), was used to assess the parenting behaviors. The scale had the followings subscales: "diet and physical activity ( PA ) Monitoring", "use food or sedentary behaviors as rewards", "pressure to eat", "restricting access to unhealthy food and sedentary behaviors", and "reinforcement" regarding adolescents' eating and PA. Five Likert-scale responses were provided for these questions (response options: never, rarely, sometimes, frequently, always or strongly disagree, disagree, neutral, agree, strongly agree). Another 1,000 data extracted randomly from the main survey was analyzed for constructed validity. Confirmatory factor analysis using LISREL 8.51 software was conducted. The description of the items as well as the results of construct validity test and reliability test were summarized in Table 3.3 and Table 3.6.

### Adolescents' pubertal status

Although it was suggested that obesity could be associated with pubertal timing (Kaplowitz, Slora, Wasserman, Pedlow, & Herman-Giddens, 2001; Tremblay & Frigon, 2005), pubertal status was not well controlled in many studies on adolescent obesity (Tsiros, Sinn, Coates, Howe, & Buckley, 2008). In this study, a self-assessment questionnaire, which required the adolescents to report their pubic hair growth, breast development (for girls), and male genital development (for boys), was used to measure the children's pubertal status. The questionnaire enabled the reliable estimation of the sexual maturation status of Chinese children (Chan, et al., 2008). The two weeks test-retest reliability of these two items in this study is 0.80 and 0.82, respectively. The internal consistency was 0.71.

### Social-demographic information

Adolescent gender and age were based on the adolescents' self-report. The background information supplied by the parents included parental education level, age, family income, and so on.

### Statistical Analysis

The correlation coefficients were calculated among adolescents' BMI, Z-BMI, dietary habits, PA level, parenting behaviors, parenting style and other related variables based on the study sample in Shantou and Ganzhou respectively. As age, gender, socioeconomic status was reported to be associated with children's weight status, dietary habits and physical activity, these factors were included in the analysis as covariates (Y. Wang, et al., 2002; Y. Wang & Zhang, 2006). Hierarchical multiple regression analysis for parenting behaviors variables and social-demographic variables predicting adolescents' Z-BMI, dietary habits and physical activity level were conducted respectively. Social-demographics variables, which could be associated with adolescents' weight status, dietary habits and physical activity level ( such as gender, age, parents' education, family income et al. ) were selected as the controlled variables in the first block in stepwise regression. Parents reported parenting behaviors variables and adolescents reported parenting behaviors variables were entered in the second block in stepwise regression respectively. Analysis of covariance ( ANCOVA ) was used to compare the scores in parenting behaviors between fathers and mothers, adjusting for adolescents' weight status, gender, and age.

## 4. 3  Results

The social-demographic information is summarized in Table 4. 1. The age of adolescents recruited in this study ranged from 10 to 15. It was found that 16. 7% of the adolescents were overweight.

**Table 4. 1   Demographic information ( N = 2, 143 )**

| | |
|---|---|
| Adolescent sex, % | |
|   Boy | 51. 4 |
|   Girl | 48. 6 |
| Adolescent age, mean ± SD, y | 12. 5 ± 0. 9 |
| Adolescent weight status, % | |
|   Underweight | 2. 4 |
|   Normal | 80. 9 |
|   Overweight | 16. 7 |
| Adolescents' BMI, mean ± SD | 18. 6 ± 2. 8 |
| Adolescent dietary habits, mean ± SD | 39. 3 ± 5. 3 |
| Adolescent physical activity, mean ± SD | 5. 1 ± 2. 8 |
| Parent sex, % | |
|   Male | 40. 4 |
|   Female | 59. 6 |
| Parent BMI, mean ± SD | 22. 2 ± 3. 0 |
| Parenting behaviors, mean ± SD | |

| | |
|---|---|
| Diet and physical activity monitoring | 19. 8 ±4. 3 |
| Use food or sedentary behaviors as rewards | 5. 4 ± 1. 8 |
| Pressure to eat | 9. 8 ±2. 1 |
| Restricting access to unhealthy food and sedentary behaviors | 15. 4 ±2. 7 |
| Reinforcement | 7. 0 ±2. 1 |
| Region, % | |
| Ganzhou | 45. 7 |
| Shantou | 54. 3 |

The correlation matrix among children's BMI, dietary habits, physical activity level, parenting behaviors, parenting styles, and parents' perception of their children's weight calculated based on the study sample in Shantou and Ganzhou were summarized in Table 4. 2, adjusting for the age, gender, family income and parents' education. As it was showed in Table 4. 2, the calculated correlation coefficients between adolescents' BMI and "diet and PA monitoring" were 0. 10 and 0. 12 in Shantou and Ganzhou respectively, both of which were statistically significant ( $p < 0.01$ ). While, the correlation coefficients between adolescents' physical activity and "reinforcement" were 0. 05 and 0. 02 in Shantou and Ganzhou respectively, both of which were not statistically significant. Since very similar correlation coefficients were found in almost all the correlation among the variables in the study sample in Shantou and Ganzhou (Table 4. 2), it was decided to combine the data in Shantou and Ganzhou together in the following data analysis.

**Table 4. 2　Correlation matrix among Adolescents' BMI, Z-BMI, dietary habits, physical activity, parenting behaviors, parenting style and parents' perception of their child's weight in Ganzhou and Shantou**

| | BMI | | Z-BMI | | Dietary habits | | Physical activity | |
|---|---|---|---|---|---|---|---|---|
| | Shantou | Ganzhou | Shantou | Ganzhou | Shantou | Ganzhou | Shantou | Ganzhou |
| Diet and PA monitoring | 0. 10 * | 0. 12 * | 0. 09 * | 0. 10 * | 0. 21 * | 0. 23 * | 0. 11 * | 0. 15 * |
| Reinforcement | 0. 01 | 0. 05 | 0. 00 | 0. 03 | 0. 10 * | 0. 09 * | 0. 05 | 0. 02 |
| Use food or sedentary behaviors as rewards | -0. 02 | 0. 01 | -0. 03 | 0. 00 | -0. 04 | -0. 02 | 0. 00 | 0. 03 |

| | | | | | | | | |
|---|---|---|---|---|---|---|---|---|
| Pressure to eat | −0.22 * | −0.18 * | −0.23 * | −0.22 * | −0.06 | −0.03 | 0.04 | 0.01 |
| Restricting access to unhealthy food and sedentary behaviors | 0.03 | 0.02 | 0.01 | 0.00 | 0.19 * | 0.23 * | 0.08 * | 0.11 * |
| Adolescents' perception of their own weight | 0.72 * | 0.68 * | 0.72 * | 0.69 * | 0.09 * | 0.10 * | −0.02 | 0.01 |
| Parents' perception of their child's weight | 0.75 * | 0.65 * | 0.74 * | 0.65 * | 0.09 * | 0.07 * | 0.00 | 0.05 |
| Paternal responsiveness | −0.01 | 0.05 | −0.02 | 0.04 | 0.20 * | 0.16 * | 0.12 * | 0.08 * |
| Maternal responsiveness | 0.00 | 0.01 | −0.01 | 0.01 | 0.18 * | 0.17 * | 0.10 * | 0.09 * |
| Paternal demandingness | −0.03 | 0.02 | −0.03 | 0.02 | 0.11 * | 0.08 * | 0.10 * | 0.08 * |
| Maternal demandingness | −0.03 | 0.01 | −0.03 | 0.01 | 0.10 * | 0.08 * | 0.10 * | 0.08 * |

Note: Age, gender, family income and parents' education were adjusted; * : $p < 0.01$

The diet and physical activity related parenting behaviors in fathers and mothers were summarized in Table 4.3. No significant difference were found between paternal and maternal parenting behaviors in "resticting access to unhealthy food and sedentary behaviors", "pressure to eat" and "reinforcement". Slight but statistical significant differences were found in "food and PA monitoring" and "use food or sedentary behaviors as rewards".

**Table 4.3  Comparison of paternal and maternal parenting behaviors, adjusting for adolescents' weight status, gender, age, parents' weight status, education level and family income**

| Parenting behaviors, mean (95% CI) | Mothers | Fathers | ANCOVA | |
|---|---|---|---|---|
| | | | F | P |
| Food and PA Monitoring | 20.5 ( 20.2 − 20.9) * * | 19.4 ( 19.0 − 19.9) * * | 14.11 | <0.01 |
| Use food or sedentary behaviors as rewards | 5.5 ( 5.3 − 5.7) * | 5.3 ( 5.1 − 5.4) * | 4.01 | <0.05 |
| Pressure to eat | 8.4 (8.3 − 8.6) | 8.3 ( 8.2 − 8.5) | 1.10 | >0.05 |
| Resticting access to unhealthy food and sedentary behaviors | 15.6 ( 15.4 − 15.8) | 15.2 (15.5) | 3.45 | >0.05 |
| Reinforcement | 7.2 (7.0 − 7.3) | 7.1 ( 6.8 − 7.3) | 0.43 | >0.05 |

* * : $P < 0.01$;  * : $P < 0.05$

The correlation among adolescents' weight status, dietary habits, physical activity, parenting behaviors were summarized in Table 4.4. Several parenting behaviors reported by adolescents and parents, including "pressure to eat" and "diet and PA monitoring", were found to be significantly related to adolescents' BMI and Z-BMI, although the correlations coefficients were not high. Moreover, it is noteworthy that the correlations coefficients between "pressure to eat" and adolescents' weight status were negative, which means that the higher adolescents' BMI, the less likely that parents may choose the feeding strategies of "pressure to eat". Furthermore, positive associations were found among "diet and PA monitoring", "reinforcement", "restricting access to unhealthy food and sedentary behaviors" and adolescents' dietary habits. In addition, statistically significant but low correlations were found between "diet and PA monitoring", "restricting access to unhealthy food and sedentary behaviors" and adolescents' physical activity level.

Table 4.4　Correlation matrix among adolescents' weight status,
dietary habits, physical activity and parenting behaviors
(data in Ganzhou and Shantou combined)

| | BMI | Z – BMI | DH | PA |
|---|---|---|---|---|
| Diet and PA monitoring | 0.10** | 0.09** | 0.21** | 0.11** |
| Reinforcement | 0.01 | 0.00 | 0.10** | 0.05 |
| Use food or sedentary behaviors as rewards | −0.02 | −0.03 | −0.04 | 0.00 |
| Pressure to eat | −0.22** | −0.23** | −0.06 | 0.04 |
| Restricting access to unhealthy food and sedentary behaviors | 0.03 | 0.01 | 0.19** | 0.08* |

Note: DH: Dietary habits; PA: Physical Activity
Age, gender, family income and parents' education were adjusted
*: $p < 0.05$; **: $p < 0.01$

Hierarchical regression models were used to predict adolescents' Z-BMI, dietary habits and physical activity respectively. As it was showed in Table 4.5, the regression model were adjusted for several social-demographic factors, including gender, age, pubertal status and parents' weight status in the first step, which explained about 9% of variance of adolescents' weight status. The data suggested that "pressure to eat" and "Diet and PA monitoring" could explain 4.2% and 1.1% of the variance of adolescents' weight status (Table 4.5). The full models using parenting behaviors could explain 14.2% of the variance of adolescents' Z-BMI.

**Table 4.5  Hierarchical regression model to predict adolescents' Z-BMI with parenting behaviors and social-demographic information**

| Predictors | B | β | 95% CI for B | Sig. | $R^2$ (unique) |
|---|---|---|---|---|---|
| Step 1 | | | | | 0.089 |
| Adolescent's gender | −0.425 | −0.113 | −0.677 — −0.173 | 0.001 | |
| Age | −0.293 | −0.135 | −0.453 — −0.134 | 0.000 | |
| Pubertal status | 0.444 | 0.223 | 0.298 – 0.590 | 0.000 | |
| Parent's weight status | 0.487 | 0.142 | 0.261 – 0.712 | 0.000 | |
| Step 2 | | | | | 0.042 |
| Pressure to eat | −0.231 | −0.274 | −0.297 — −0.165 | 0.000 | |
| Step 3 | | | | | 0.011 |
| Diet and PA monitoring | 0.133 | 0.123 | 0.048 – 0.217 | 0.002 | |

Model $R^2$: 0.143; Final multiple R = 0.378, P < 0.01

Note: Only variables with statistic significant in the model were presented.

The results of hierarchical regression for the adolescents' dietary habits predication were summarized in Table 4.6. In the first step, gender and age accounted for about 4% of the variability. For the parents reported parenting behaviors, "parents' diet and PA monitoring" and "resticting access to unhealthy food and sedentary behaviors" accounted for only 3.9% and 0.9% of variability respectively (Table 4.6). This model could only explain 9% of the variance of adolescents' dietary habits.

**Table 4. 6  Hierarchical regression model to predict adolescents' dietary habits with parenting behaviors and social-demographic information**

| Predictors | B | β | 95% CI for B | Sig. | $R^2$ (unique) |
|---|---|---|---|---|---|
| Step 1 | | | | | 0. 046 |
| Adolescent's gender | 1. 470 | 0. 371 | 0. 742 – 2. 198 | 0. 000 | |
| Step 2 | | | | | 0. 039 |
| Diet and PA monitoring | 0. 181 | 0. 147 | 0. 083 – 0. 279 | 0. 000 | |
| Step 3 | | | | | 0. 009 |
| Resticting access to unhealthy food and sedentary behaviors | 0. 225 | 0. 117 | 0. 076 – 0. 374 | 0. 003 | |

Model $R^2$: 0. 090; Final multiple R = 0. 300, P < 0. 01

Note: Only variables with statistic significant in the model were presented.

For the predication of adolescents' physical activity, several social-demographic variables including gender, father's education level and family income were found to be associated with adolescents' physical activity, explaining nearly 13% of the variability (Table 4. 7). The results of regression revealed that "parents' diet and PA monitoring" may explain 1. 3% of the variance of adolescents' PA. The percentage of the variance of adolescents' PA could be explained by the model was only 14. 0%.

**Table 4. 7  Hierarchical regression model to predict adolescents' physical activity with parenting behaviors and social-demographic information**

| Predictors | B | β | 95% CI for B | Sig. | $R^2$ (unique) |
|---|---|---|---|---|---|
| Step 1 | | | | | 0. 127 |
| Adolescent's gender | – 1. 506 | – 0. 301 | – 1. 845— – 1. 167 | 0. 000 | |
| Father's education level | 0. 394 | 0. 140 | 0. 119 – 0. 669 | 0. 005 | |
| Family income | 0. 375 | 0. 086 | 0. 077 – 0. 699 | 0. 014 | |
| Step 2 | | | | | 0. 013 |
| Parents' diet and PA monitoring | 0. 069 | 0. 020 | 0. 029 – 0. 109 | 0. 001 | |

Model $R^2$: 0. 140; Final multiple R = 0. 374, P < 0. 01

Note: Only variables with statistic significant in the model were presented.

## 4. 4  Discussion and conclusion

The present study is one of the few studies investigating the association between parenting behaviors and adolescent obesity in China. The data of this study revealed that several parenting behaviors were significantly correlated to adolescents' BMI, dietary habits and physical activity, although only low percentage of the variances of adolescents' weight status, dietary habits and PA could be explained by these parenting behaviors.

"Pressure to eat" is one of frequently used parents' feeding behaviors, which means encouraging or forcing children to eat. Previous studies suggested that this type of parenting behaviors may have long term effects on children's food intake and weight status (Clark, et al., 2007). For instance, "pressure to eat" was found to be associated with higher fruit and vegetable intake (Bourcier, et al., 2003). A cross-sectional study showed that "pressure to eat" was negative related to children's weight status (Spruijt-Metz, et al., 2002). Another longitudinal study revealed that parents always choose their feeding strategy based on their children's weight status. It was found out that, towards thinner children, parents were found to be more likely to use the behaviors of "pressure to eat" but less likely to use "restriction" strategies (Lee, Mitchell, Smiciklas-Wright, & Birch, 2001). The result of this study also confirmed these findings. The data of this study showed that "pressure to eat" was negatively related to adolescents' BMI ($r = -0.22$, $p < 0.01$) and Z – BMI ($r = -0.23$, $p < 0.01$). In addition, the data of this study showed that the parenting behavior of "pressure to eat" could explain 4. 2% the variance of adolescents' weight status. The results of another study showed that "pressure to eat" and parents' concern for their children' weight status were found to explain 15% of the variance of children's total fat mass (Spruijt-Metz, et al., 2002). As two kinds of parenting behaviors were included in the same block in Spruijt-Mets's regression model, it may not be able to compare the data in Spruijt-Mets's study and ours. However, both of the studies suggested that "pressure to eat" is significantly associated with children's weight status.

Several parents' feeding behaviors including food restriction and using food as rewards were found to be associated with children's food intake (Rhee, 2008). For instance, adverse effects of restricting access to food on children's food intake were reported. In turns, children's weight status may also influence parental restriction (Fisher & Birch, 1999a). The present study found that parents' restriction feeding behaviors were positively correlated to adolescents' dietary habits. Moreover, the results of hierarchical regression also indicated that "resticting access to unhealthy food and sedentary behaviors" was one of the significant predictors for adolescents' dietary habits. In addition, the data revealed the correlation between "diet and PA monitoring" and adolescents' dietary intake as well, which was consistent to the findings from previous studies (Lindsay, et al., 2006; Rhee, 2008), although it was noteworthy that the percentage of variability of adolescents' dietary habits explained by other parenting behaviors was not high.

Sufficient physical activity is regarded as one of the key components in weight control programs (Jakicic & Otto, 2005). Research suggested that parenting behaviors may influence their children's physical activity level. For instance, it was found that when compared with the children of physical inactive parents, the children of active parents had higher odds ratio of being active (Moore, et al., 1991). It was also reported that the children received more parental support for sports participation were more physically active than the ones received less support (O'Loughlin, et al., 1999). However, inconsistent results were found in several studies. It was reported that girls' physical activity were related to parents reported support but not associated with girls' perception of parent's support for physical activity (Adkins, et al., 2004). Another study revealed that parent support significantly correlated with adolescent self-reported physical activities, but not related to the adolescents' physical activity measured by accelerometers (Prochaska, et al., 2002). The results of the present study showed that "PA monitoring" and "restricting access to sedentary behaviors" were significantly associated with adolescents' physical activity. However, hierarchical model showed that parenting behaviors could only explain very low percentage of the variance of adolescents' physical activity. The data of present study indicated that parenting behaviors could be weakly but statistically significant related to adolescents' physical activity.

In addition, we failed to find large differences between paternal and maternal parenting behaviors in this study, although slight but significant differences were found in several parenting behaviors. For hundreds years, Chinese families were influenced by Confucian ideas, in which women had low status in the household (S. W. K. Yu & Chau, 1997). However, the patriarchy of Chinese family was challenged since the implementation of one-child policy in 1979. Recent study indicated that the one-child policy is undermining patrilineal norms in China and the positions of women are improved significantly (Deutsch, 2006). Therefore, the slight differences in parenting behaviors in Chinese fathers and mothers could be partly explained by the promotion of gender equality in family during the past 3 decades.

Since the single-child family planning program was implemented in the 1970s in mainland China, millions of Chinese's parenting behaviors and parenting style was modified (Jing, 1994). Many Chinese children were treated like a little emperor or empress at home by their parents, which could be significantly different from traditional Chinese parenting style. For instance, parents always like to add some dishes to their children to express their love to children. It was reported that 56.0% parents often reminded their children to eat some food they regarded as healthy food, and 7.7% parents often forced their children to eat these food (W. J. Ma, et al., 2001). The data of this study also indicated that "pressure to eat" was also frequently used by Chinese parents, which seems not consistent with the traditional "authoritarian" and "controlling" parenting in China. As this feeding strategy could influence children's own capability to regulate calories intake, "pressure to eat" may contribute to energy over-consumption and childhood obesity. The findings suggest that not only parenting behaviors but also parents' beliefs should be considered in the intervention.

There are several limitations in the present study that need to be clarified. First of all, as the study design of present study is cross sectional study, the direction of cause and effect could not be determined. Other limitations may include the self-report nature of the data and non-national representative sample. There were also several strengths in this study which include large sample size and well developed questionnaires with acceptable validity and reliability.

In conclusion, it was successfully demonstrated in the present study that adolescents' weight status, dietary habits and physical activity were statistically significant but weakly associated with some parenting behaviors, including "pressure to eat", "diet and physical activity monitoring", "restricting access to unhealthy food and sedentary behaviors" and some other parenting behaviors. However, we failed to find large differences in parenting behaviors between Chinese fathers and mothers.

# CHAPTER 5   PARENTS' PERCEPTIONS OF THEIR CHILDREN's WEIGHTS AND THEIR RELATION TO PARENTING BEHAVIORS

## 5. 1   Introduction

Childhood obesity is a growing epidemic worldwide. The incidence of childhood obesity has increased in most developed and developing countries. In China, as the nutritional problems shift from malnutrition to overnutrition in children and adolescents ( Y. Wang, et al. , 2002 ), the prevalence of obese children aged 2 to 6 years increased from 1. 5% to 12. 6% , and the prevalence of overweight individuals increased from 14. 6% to 28. 6% in urban areas of China from 1989 to 1997 ( Luo & Hu  2002 ).

Modifications of some eating habits and physical activities were recommended to the children and the parents to help prevent excessive weight gain of the children ( Barlow & the Expert Committee, 2007 ). Since parents play a key role in shaping their children's eating habits and inclination to do physical activities ( Rhee, 2008 ), parents' readiness and willingness to modify their parenting behaviors or parenting styles may be important steps toward helping their children lose weight. The Health Belief Model suggested that one of the key factors that determine individuals' health-related behaviors is their perception of their susceptibility to a particular health problem ( Elder, Ayala, & Harris, 1999; Janz & Becker, 1984; Rhee, 2008 ). Therefore, parents may not be too willing to change their behaviors until they recognize the weight problems of their children. Recent studies also proved the correlation between parental perception of children's weights and the parents' readiness to help their children lose weight (Rhee, et al. , 2005).

Unfortunately, recent European and American studies have reported high percentages of parental misconception of their children's weight (Eckstein, et al. , 2006; Etelson, et al. , 2003; Ward, 2008). For instance, a cross-sectional survey in the United States showed that 95% of obese mothers believed that their children were overweight. However, nearly 80% of the mothers failed to perceive their overweight children as overweight (Baughcum, et al. , 2000). The results of a study in Germany revealed that only 40.3% of the mothers correctly recognized their children's weight (Warschburger & Kroller, 2009). The data of Chinese parents' perception of their child's weight was reported by several cross-sectional surveys in mainland China (Shi, et al. , 2007; Xie, et al. , 2006). It was found that about 22% of the parents regarded their children as underweight even if their children had normal weights. Meanwhile, of the overweight children, 23% were perceived by their parents as having normal weights (Shi, et al. , 2007).

The factors that may influence parents' perceptions of their children's weights had been widely discussed in recent studies. Children's and parents' characteristics, including children's weights, children's ages, children's sex, parents' weights, parental education level, and family incomes had been reported to be associated with parental perceptions of their children's weights (Baughcum, et al. , 2000; Campbell, Williams, Hampton, & Wake, 2006; Huang, et al. , 2007; Warschburger & Kroller, 2009). However, few studies had investigated the direct relationship between parental perception of children's weights and parenting behaviors to promote healthy dietary and physical activity habits (Hodges, 2003), even if some studies had already determined a correlation between parenting behaviors and the development of childhood obesity (Birch & Fisher, 1998; Faith, Scanlon, et al. , 2004; Rhee, 2008). In addition, although Chinese adolescents' and parents' weight perceptions were reported by several studies (Shi, et al. , 2007; Xie, et al. , 2006; Xie, et al. , 2003), the studies concentrated on adolescents' own weight perceptions and weight satisfaction. There have not been substantial reports on Chinese parents' perceptions of their children's weights. Therefore, the purpose of this study is to examine Chinese parents' perceptions of their adolescent children's weights and to explore the parenting behaviors associated with these perceptions.

## 5.2 Methods

### Study population and procedure

The study population of present study was the adolescents and their parents in urban areas of southern China, due to much higher prevalence of obesity in the urban areas as compared with rural areas (Luo & Hu, 2002). As improved economic and social conditions was found to be an important factor that may lead to Chinese's increased nutrient-dense and energy-dense food intake, sedentary lifestyle and weight status (Y. Wang, et al., 2002), it was decided to recruited our participants from a developed city and an underdeveloped city in southern China. Stratified random sampling was applied in the present study, in which a city (Shantou) in developed area and a city (Ganzhou) in underdeveloped area were chosen. Shantou, one of the original Special Economic Zones of China established in the 1980s, is one of the developed regions in southern China. The Gross Domestic Product (GDP) per capita in Shantou was 20, 279 RMB (Shantou municipal bureau of statistics, 2010). Ganzhou, one of the old revolutionary base areas in China, is an underdeveloped inland city located in southern China. The GDP per capita in Ganzhou was 9, 391 RMB (Ganzhou municipal bureau of statistics, 2010). Adolescents and their parents were randomly recruited from grade 1 and grade 2 of secondary schools in Ganzhou and Shantou respectively. For example, in Ganzhou, there are two districts. In the present study, a key secondary school and an ordinary secondary school was randomly chosen in each district. 4 – 6 classes in each school (2 – 3 classes in each grade) were randomly drawn in the investigation. The same sampling strategy was applied in Shantou. Exclusion criteria for adolescents was using medications that may influence weight gain or loss, and a diagnosis of physical or developmental disability or chronic illness. From April to May 2009, 2, 162 pairs of adolescents and parents participated in the present survey (Ganzhou: 1,179 pairs; Shantou: 1,106 pairs). There were 19 adolescents who had physical disability or received medications that influence their weight status were excluded from the analysis. 274 parents did not send the questionnaire back. Consequently, 2,143 adolescents and 1,869 their parents were finally included in the data analysis.

During the survey, adolescents aged 10 to 15 years were invited to complete an anthropometric test for body weight and height, and were asked to fill out questionnaires inside a classroom with the assistance of an investigator. The adolescents were also asked to take home the "questionnaires for parents", to ask either their mothers or fathers to fill out the questionnaires, and to give these back to the survey conductors. Souvenirs were given to the participants as compliments.

Other than the participants in the main survey, 127 pairs (Ganzhou: 62 pairs, Shantou: 65 pairs) were invited to participate in a pilot study beforehand. During the pilot study, adolescents and their parents were required to complete the questionnaires twice with two weeks apart. The test-retest reliability of each item and internal consistency was determined by intraclass correlation coefficient (ICC) and Cronbach's alpha respectively.

Signed informed consent was obtained from all participants (including adolescents and parents) prior to the survey. The adolescents and their parents were briefly introduced that they need to provide some information about their children's health status and were highly encouraged to honestly report what they really think and what they did. In the instruction of the questionnaire, both adolescents and parents were clearly informed that there is no right or wrong answers for each item and the questionnaire is anonymous. Formal approval was granted from the Chinese University of Hong Kong Research Ethics Committee.

## Main study measures

### Adolescent weight status

An adolescent's body weight to the nearest 0.1 kg was measured with minimal clothing and without shoes using a measuring scale. An adolescent's body height to the nearest 0. 5 cm was taken using a stadiometer. An adolescent's body mass index ( BMI ) was calculated as his weight in kilograms divided by the square of his height in meters, and was categorized either as underweight ( thinness, BMI-for-age $< -2$ SD), normal or, overweight ( BMI-for-age $> 1$ SD) based on the international growth standards for school-aged children and adolescents updated by the World Health Organization ( WHO) ( Butte, et al. , 2007; De Onis, et al. , 2007).

### Parent weight status

The BMIs of parents were recorded based on their self-reported heights and weights, as it is not feasible to measure parents' height and weight in the present study. Validity of self-reported heights and weights of adults were well reported ( Bolton-Smith, et al. , 2000; Wada, et al. , 2005). Pearson's r between self-reported BMI and measured BMI was 0. 943 and 0. 950 for men and women, respectively ( Wada, et al. , 2005). According to the BMI reference for screening overweight and obesity among Chinese adults, parental BMIs were categorized either as non-overweight ( BMI $< 24$ kg/$m^2$ ) or overweight ( 24 kg/$m^2$ $\leqslant$ BMI $< 28$ kg/$m^2$ ), or obese ( BMI $\geqslant 28$ kg/$m^2$ ) ( Zhou & Cooperative Meta-Analysis Group of the Working Group on Obesity in China, 2002).

### Parental perceptions of their children's weights

To assess the parents' perceptions of their children's weights, parents were asked to report their children's weights subjectively by giving any one of the five possible answers: " very underweight ", " slightly underweight ", " normal ", " slightly overweight ", and " very overweight ". To aid in the analysis, the perception levels of the subjects were further categorized into either " underweight " ( " very underweight " or " slightly underweight " ), " normal " ( " normal " ), or " overweight " ( " slightly overweight " or " very overweight " ) group. The test-retest reliability of this item was 0. 88.

### Adolescents' perceptions of their own weights

Figure drawings developed by Collins were used to examine adolescents' perceptions of their weights ( Collins, 1991 ). The drawings were consisted of seven figures, whose descriptions ranged from very thin to very obese. In this study, adolescents were instructed to choose any one of the seven figures to answer the following question: "Which picture looks the most like how you look?" The test-retest reliability of this item based on Grade 1 – 3 children with 3 days internal was 0. 71 (Collins, 1991). The results of reliability test in current study showed that the test-retest reliability was 0. 92. To aid in the analysis, the perception levels of the subjects were further categorized into "underweight", "normal", or "overweight" groups according to the classification method used in a previous study (Warschburger & Kroller, 2009). The adolescents who selected the thinnest 2 figures were categorized as "underweight"; the ones selected the next 3 figures were categorized as "normal" and the ones selected the heaviest 2 figures were categorized as "overweight". The adolescent's/parents' weight perceptions, depending on consistency of these to the actual weights, were defined either as "correct" or "incorrect".

**Parenting behaviors**

An 17 – item, five-point Likert-type scale, which was modified and translated based on the questionnaires used in previous studies (Arredondo, et al. , 2006; O'Connor, et al. , 2010), was used to assess the parenting behaviors. The scale had the followings subscales: "diet and physical activity (PA) Monitoring", "use food or sedentary behaviors as rewards", "pressure to eat", "restricting access to unhealthy food and sedentary behaviors", and "reinforcement" regarding adolescents' eating and PA. Five Likert-scale responses were provided for these questions (response options: never, rarely, sometimes, frequently, always or strongly disagree, disagree, neutral, agree, strongly agree). Another data from the main survey was analyzed for construct validity. Confirmatory factor analysis using LISREL 8. 51 software was conducted. The description of the items as well as the results of construct validity test and reliability test were summarized in Table 3. 3 and Table 3. 6.

**Others**

Adolescents' gender and age were recorded based on the adolescents' own reports. Background information supplied by the parents included parental education level, age, and family income, among others.

### Data analysis

The agreement of the parents' (adolescents') weight perceptions with the adolescents' actual weights were tested using Kappa statistics. Multinomial logistic regression was used to predict the risk factors that influence the accuracy of the parents' perception of their adolescents' weights. Analysis of covariance (ANCOVA) was used to compare the scores in parenting behaviors among parents with accurate perceptions and those who have misconceptions of their children's weights. As age, gender, socioeconomic status was reported to be associated with children's weight status, these factors were included in the analysis as covariates (Y. Wang, et al., 2002; Y. Wang & Zhang, 2006).

## 5. 3   Results

A total of 2, 143 adolescents and 1, 869 their parents were included in this study. The demographic information is summarized in Table 5. 1.

**Table 5. 1   Demographic information ( N = 2, 143 )**

| | |
|---|---|
| Adolescent sex, % | |
|   Boy | 51. 4 |
|   Girl | 48. 6 |
| Adolescent age, mean ± SD, y | 12. 5 ± 0. 9 |
| Adolescent weight status, % | |
|   Underweight | 2. 4 |
|   Normal | 80. 9 |
|   Overweight | 16. 7 |
| Adolescents' BMI, mean ± SD | 18. 6 ± 2. 8 |
| Adolescent dietary habits, mean ± SD | 39. 3 ± 5. 3 |
| Adolescent physical activity, mean ± SD | 5. 1 ± 2. 8 |
| Parent sex, % | |
|   Male | 40. 4 |
|   Female | 59. 6 |
| Parent BMI, mean ± SD | 22. 2 ± 3. 0 |
| Parenting behaviors, mean ± SD | |
|   Diet and physical activity monitoring | 19. 8 ± 4. 3 |

| | |
|---|---|
| Use food or sedentary behaviors as rewards | 5.4 ± 1.8 |
| Pressure to eat | 9.8 ± 2.1 |
| Restricting access to unhealthy food and sedentary behaviors | 15.4 ± 2.7 |
| Reinforcement | 7.0 ± 2.1 |
| Region, % | |
| Ganzhou | 45.7 |
| Shantou | 54.3 |

The data of this study showed about two out of five parents mistakenly identified their children's weight, while nearly three out of five adolescents did not correctly report their weights. As shown in Table 5.2, there was only a minimal agreement between the adolescents' BMIs and their parents' perception of their children's weights ( Kappa = 0.221, p < 0.01 ). About 40% of parents of overweight adolescents believed that their children had normal weights or were underweight. Of the parents, 42.2% regarded their normal-weight children as underweight. Poor agreement was also found between the adolescents' actual BMIs and their perceptions of their own weights ( Kappa = 0.167, p < 0.01 ). Nearly 30% of the overweight adolescents classified themselves either as adolescents with normal weights or as underweight. Moreover, 55.0% of normal-weight adolescents considered themselves "underweight".

**Table 5.2  The agreement of the adolescents' BMI category with their parents' and the adolescents' weight perception**

| | Adolescents' BMI category ( N, % ) | | | kappa |
|---|---|---|---|---|
| | underweight | normal | overweight | |
| Parental perception | | | | 0.221 |
| Underweight | 44(91.7) | 626(42.2) | 6(1.9) | |
| normal | 2(4.2) | 802(54.1) | 120(38.5) | |
| overweight | 2(4.2) | 55(3.7) | 186(59.6) | |
| Adolescents' perception | | | | 0.167 |
| Underweight | 44(84.6) | 949(55.0) | 21(5.9) | |
| normal | 8(15.4) | 635(36.8) | 90(25.3) | |
| overweight | 0(0) | 141(8.2) | 245(68.8) | |

Note: 10 adolescents and 26 parents were excluded from the analysis because of incomplete data about them

The data of this study showed that several factors could be associated with parental weight perception (Table 5.3). It was learned that Chinese parents were more likely to incorrectly identify a boy's weight than a girl's weight ( OR = 1.61, 95% CI 1.29 – 2.01). Compared with fathers, mothers were less likely to have wrong perceptions about their children's weight ( OR = 0.80, 95% CI: 0.64 – 1.00). The results of the logistic regression also suggested that there was a correlation between parental perception of their children's weights and the adolescents' own perception of their weights. Unlike the parents whose children failed to correctly perceive their own weights, the parents whose children correctly reported their weights had better ability to recognize their children's weights ( OR = 0.30, 95% CI: 0.24 – 0.38 ). For the other adolescents' and parental characteristics, no significant independent association was found.

Table 5.3　Odds ratio for parental ability to incorrectly ( versus correctly )
identify their children's weight according to selected variables

|  |  | Adjusted OR (95% CI) |
|---|---|---|
| Adolescents' Gender | Girl | Reference |
|  | Boy | 1.61 (1.29 – 2.01) * * |
| Adolescents' weight perception | Incorrect | Reference |
|  | correct | 0.30 (0.24 – 0.38) * * |
| Parents' gender | father | Reference |
|  | Mother | 0.80 (0.64 – 1.00) * |
| Number of children in the family | 1 | Reference |
|  | ≥2 | 0.99 (0.72 – 1.35) |
| Parents' weight status | Normal | Reference |
|  | overweight | 0.98 (0.75 – 1.28) |
|  | obesity | 0.66 (0.37 – 1.20) |
| Parents' education | Junior middle school or lower | Reference |
|  | Senior high school | 0.94 (0.70 – 1.27) |
|  | College or higher | 0.70 (0.53 – 1.10) |
| Family income | Low | Reference |
|  | Middle | 0.94 (0.73 – 1.19) |
|  | High | 0.88 (0.48 – 1.60) |
| Location | Ganzhou | Reference |
|  | Shantou | 1.18 (0.86 – 1.62) |

Adjusted for adolescents' age and weights.

* : P < .05; * * : P < .01

Parenting behaviors, which could be associated with the development of childhood obesity, were compared between the parents who correctly and incorrectly perceived their children's weights, using ANCOVA test (adjusting for adolescents' weight status, gender, and age) (Table 5.4). The data of this study suggest that indeed, there are differences between the parents with correct perception of their children's weights and those with incorrect perception. Compared with the parents who have wrong perceptions of their children's weights, the parents who have correct perception of their children's weights got higher scores in monitoring their adolescents' dietary and physical activities ($p < .01$), and gave more positive reinforcement to their children for manifesting healthy behaviors ($p < .05$). Parents with incorrect perception of their children's weights were more likely to select the feeding strategy of "pressure to eat" ($p < .01$) compared to parents with correct perception. However, no significant difference were found in "use food or sedentary behaviors as rewards" and "restricting access to unhealthy food and sedentary behaviors" between parents with correct and incorrect perception.

**Table 5.4  Comparison of Parenting Behaviors of Parents With Correct and Incorrect Perception of Their Children's Weight**

| | Score in parenting behaviors Mean (95% CI) | | ANCOVA Test | | |
| --- | --- | --- | --- | --- | --- |
| | Correct | Incorrect | F | p | Cohen's $d$ |
| Food and PA monitoring | 20.38 (20.05 – 20.71) | 19.52 (19.15 – 19.89) | 11.93 | 0.001 | 0.20 |
| Use food or sedentary behaviors as rewards | 5.62 (5.48 – 5.76) | 5.52 (5.36 – 5.67) | 0.58 | 0.447 | 0.06 |
| Pressure to eat | 9.69 (9.53 – 9.86) | 10.12 (10.01 – 10.38) | 20.26 | 0.000 | 0.21 |
| Restricting access to unhealthy food and sedentary behaviors | 15.56 (15.34 – 15.78) | 15.35 (15.10 – 15.59) | 1.62 | 0.204 | 0.08 |
| Reinforcement | 7.20 (7.04 – 7.36) | 6.95 (6.77 – 7.13) | 4.05 | 0.044 | 0.12 |

Note: adolescents' weight, gender and age were adjusted.

## 5. 4 Discussion and conclusion

The results of this study show that 16. 7% of the adolescents are overweight, and over a quarter of the parents are overweight or obese. Childhood obesity has become an emerging major public health problem in China ( Ji & Working Group on Obesity in China, 2005) although its prevalence has not yet reached the levels seen in other developed countries. This study shows a slight agreement between parental perception of their children's weights and the adolescents' actual weights. A higher percentage of misconception of the children's weight in Chinese parents was found ( Table 2) compared with data in 2002 ( Shi, et al. , 2007). This could be caused by time-varying difference and the difference in research methods ( sampling design and measurement instruments). Data from the present survey revealed that only 56% of the parents correctly reported their children's weights. Similar results were reported by other studies. The results of a study conducted in the US showed that only 60% of the respondent mothers accurately assessed the weights of their children ( Boutelle, Fulkerson, Neumark-Sztainer, & Story, 2004). This study shows that Chinese parents are not better at identifying their children's weights although a race/ethnicity difference in the accuracy of parental perception of their children's weight was reported ( Boutelle, et al. , 2004). In addition, the WHO growth reference where the BMI values at + 1 SD are 25. 4 kg/m$^2$ for boys and 25. 0 kg/m$^2$ for girls at 19 years old ( De Onis, et al. , 2007) was used in the present study. This standard is linked to the overweight cut-off points ( 25 kg/m$^2$ ) , and higher than the overweight standard for Chinese ( 24 kg/ m$^2$ ) ( Zhou & Cooperative Meta-Analysis Group of the Working Group on Obesity in China, 2002). Therefore, the prevalence of parents' misclassification of their children's weight could be even higher if a lower standard for overweight is applied.

Parental assessment of the weights of their children was reported to be associated with the characteristics of the parents themselves, as well as their children ( Huang, et al. , 2007). The results of this study reveal that parental perceptions of their children's weights are associated with gender, and the latter's perceptions of their own weights. Overweight daughters are more likely to elicit maternal concern (Campbell, et al., 2006; Maynard, Galuska, Blanck, & Serdula, 2003) compared with overweight sons. Chinese parents are also more likely to mistakenly perceive their sons' weights than their daughters'. Mothers were also found to have better ability to discriminate their children's weights. The main reason for this gender difference could be related to social values (Campbell, et al., 2006). For instance, girls with slender and graceful stature are favorably perceived by society, while overweight boys are sometimes regarded as strong and healthy rather than obese. Therefore, Chinese parents are more sensitive to weight issues concerning their daughters than their sons, similar to parents from the US and Australia (Campbell, et al., 2006; Maynard, et al., 2003).

The reasons for parents' misclassification of their children's' weights are still not determined. It may be caused by parents' weak recognition of their children's true weights, lack of understanding of the definition of the words "overweight" and "obesity," and emotional factors such as parents' unwillingness to admit that their children are overweight or obese (Maynard, et al., 2003). A qualitative study revealed that low income US mothers preferred to describe their overweight children as thick or solid rather than overweight or obese (Jain, et al., 2001). A recent study showed that socioeconomic status is not associated with maternal classification of their own children's weight but with the identification of overweight in unrelated children (Warschburger & Kroller, 2009). Therefore, mothers' perception of their own children may be more influenced by emotional factors than "cognitive" factors such as knowledge about obesity and body image, which could be related to educational level. The study shows that parental perceptions of their children's weights are associated with gender, but not associated with the parents' education level and family income. Similarly, it could be explained that the parents' perception of their children's weight may be mainly caused by emotional factors, which could be related to the parents' and adolescent gender, rather than factors like education level, family income, and number of children in the family. However, the present study could not confirm this assumption. Further studies are needed to investigate the reasons.

The Health Belief Model suggests that the primary motivation to behavior modification in weight management is the level of perceived threat or risk of obesity ( Daddario, 2007). Therefore, addressing misconceptions of children and their parents on the children's weights may be an important first step to weight management. Previous studies suggested that underestimating children's weights by their parents and by the children themselves were associated with poorer diet behaviors and increase in the perceived barriers to the observation of a healthy diet or desire to exercise ( Skinner, Weinberger, Mulvaney, Schlundt, & Rothman, 2008 ). Moreover, feedback on children's and adolescent's risk for overweight problem is recommended to increase parents' risk awareness and willingness to modify their parenting behaviors ( Warschburger & Kroller, 2009 ). A study examined the psychological impact of a school-based weight-screening intervention that gave feedback to parents. The results showed that feedback did not influence changes in child feeding among parents of healthy-weight children. However, parents of overweight girls imposed more dietary restrictions on their daughters ( Grimmett, Croker, Carnell, & Wardle, 2008 ). Another cross-sectional study showed that accurate classification of an overweight child may not translate into helpful behaviors and may lead to unhealthy behaviors such as encouragement to diet ( Neumark-Sztainer, Wall, Story, & van den Berg, 2008 ). Several parenting behaviors including " food and PA monitoring," "pressure to eat," and "reinforcement" were found to be associated with parental perceptions of their children's weight in the current study. These parenting behaviors have been proven to be associated with childhood obesity ( Birch & Fisher, 1998; Rhee, 2008 ). For instance, some studies indicated that parents' "pressure to eat" strategy correlates with children's caloric intake ( Drucker, Hammer, Agras, & Bryson, 1999) and total fat mass ( Spruijt-Metz, Lindquist, Birch, Fisher, & Goran, 2002 ). The present study reveals that parents with correct perception of their children's weight are associated with lower frequency of using the strategy of 'pressure to eat," compared with the parents with incorrect perception. Although only a small effect is found in the current study, the differences should not be ignored (Pedersen, 2003). The results still indicate that accurate classification of children's weights may be related to positive parenting behaviors, which could benefit childhood obesity prevention.

The results of this study also show the correlation between adolescents' perceptions of their own weights and their parents' perception. Another study based on 718 children and their parents also indicated that parents' judgment of adolescents' weights may affect their children's perceptions of their own weights (Huang, Donohue, Becerra, & Xu, 2009). The results of these studies suggest that parental perception of their children's weight is associated with parenting behaviors as well as adolescents' perception of their own weight, both of which may contribute to the development of adolescent obesity.

Several limitations need to be acknowledged and addressed regarding the present study. One is that the BMI rather than body fat was used to classify adolescents' weights. Although using BMI-for-age percentiles for screening overweight and obese children was effective (Ji & Working Group on Obesity in China, 2005; Mei, et al. , 2002), there might have been mistakes in the weight classifications in this study because the BMI is not a direct measurement of body fat. Second, Collins' drawings, which were used to classify adolescents' perception of their own weight, are not based on individuals of a specific BMI range. The format and style of Collins'drawings are similar to the ones developed by Warschburger and Kroller based on specific preschool-aged children's BMI percentile (2009). The classification method used in Warschburger and Kroller's study was then applied in the current study, although it is a limitation that needs to be acknowledged. The results could also not be applied to all Chinese in the world because the sample was drawn only from limited urban areas in Southern China. Other limitations that should be considered in interpreting the results include the "self-report" nature of certain data and the cross-sectional study design.

The survey, in spite of its limitations, still successfully demonstrates that misconceptions about children's weights are prevalent among Chinese parents. The accuracy of parental perception of children's weights could be associated with gender, and the adolescents' perceptions of their own weights. The association between parents' perception of their children's weight and parenting behaviors suggests that the accurate classification of children's weights could help prevent childhood obesity.

# CHAPTER 6　Parenting Style as a Moderator of Association Between Parenting behaviors and Adolescent's Weight Status

## 6.1　Introduction

Childhood obesity is a public health issue that is becoming an increasingly important problem in developed countries (Lehingue, 1999; Ogden, Flegal, Carroll, & Johnson, 2002). In the past 10 years, the obesity epidemic among children and adolescents has also been growing rapidly in China (Ji & Working Group on Obesity in China, 2005). Parents could play key roles in the development and prevention of childhood obesity. It was reported that childhood obesity could be associated with parenting behaviors (Clark, et al., 2007). For instance, parental feeding behavior may influence the development of children's eating habits and food preference, their ability to regulate energy intake, and ultimately their weight status (Nguyen, et al., 1996). In addition, recent research revealed that children's weight problem could be related to their parents' parenting style (Rhee, et al., 2006).

Parenting style is defined as "a constellation of attitudes toward the child, which are communicated to him or her, and which, taken together, create an emotional climate in which the parent's behaviors are expressed" (Darling & Steinberg, 1993). The most widely used theory of parenting style was firstly established in 1970s, in which parenting styles were conceptualized based on the amount and quality of two underlying dimensions: demandingness and responsiveness (Baumrind, 1971). According to the two dimensions, parenting style can be categorized into 4 main styles ( authoritative, authoritarian, permissive and neglectful). Parenting style could be very important in childhood obesity prevention because it provides the environmental and emotional context for children's growth, as well as the context in which specific parenting behaviors are expressed ( Rhee, 2008). Several studies investigated the relationship between parenting style and childhood obesity. It was found that children of authoritarian, permissive, and neglectful mothers had an increased risk of being overweight ( Rhee, et al. , 2006 ). The results of a longitudinal study in Australia also indicated that fathers' parenting styles may be related to the risk for childhood obesity ( Wake, et al. , 2007 ). Furthermore, a cross-sectional study based on 163 Chinese children ( aged 8 to 10 years ) and their mothers also revealed a positive relationship between democratic parenting and the children's BMI ( J. L. Chen & Kennedy, 2004 ). However, the mechanism of how parenting style influence children's weight status is still not clear.

In addition, cultural difference in parenting style should be considered. Although the the theory of parenting style established by Baumrind ( 1971 ) was widely applied in the studies on Chinese population ( X. Y. Chen, et al. , 1997; Pong, et al. , 2009; Porter, et al. , 2005 ), it was suggested that Chinese parents maybe accustomed to being authoritative and authoritarian ( Xu, et al. , 2005 ). Moreover, since there is no standard cut-off points for the scales to measure parenting style, the four parenting styles are categorized based on a relative criterion ( such as median ), which would cause different cut-off points in different populations. Therefore, the continuous measures of responsiveness and demandingness rather than the four parenting style categories maybe more appropriate for Chinese parents.

Darling & Steinberg ( 1993 ) postulated parenting style functions as a moderator of the effects of parenting practices on adolescents' outcomes. According to this contextual model of parenting style, the effect of parenting behaviors on adolescents' weight status could be enhanced by parenting style. Van der Horst et al. ( 2007 ) confirmed that parenting style could moderate the relationship between parenting practices and children's sugar-sweetened beverage consumption. However, few studies investigated such moderating effects in the association between the parenting behaviors and children's weight status.

Therefore, based on the contextual model of parenting style, the purpose of this study is to examine whether the association between parenting behaviors and adolescents' outcome (dietary habits, physical activity and weight status) is moderated by parenting style.

## 6.2 Methods

### Study population and procedure

The study population of present study was the adolescents and their parents in urban areas of southern China, due to much higher prevalence of obesity in the urban areas as compared with rural areas (Luo & Hu, 2002). Stratified random sampling was applied in the present study, in which a city (Shantou) in developed area and a city (Ganzhou) in underdeveloped area were chosen. Adolescents and their parents were randomly recruited from grade 1 (12 ± 1 years) and grade 2 (13 ± 1 years) of secondary schools in Ganzhou and Shantou respectively. In the present study, two districts were randomly selected in each city. A key secondary school and an regular secondary school was randomly chosen in each district. 4 – 6 classes in each school (2 – 3 classes in each grade) were randomly drawn in the investigation. From April to May 2009, 2, 162 Parent-adolescent dyads participated in the present survey (Ganzhou: 1, 179 dyads; Shantou: 1, 106 dyads). Over 99% participants were Han Chinese. There were 19 adolescents who had physical disability or received medications that influence their weight status were excluded from the analysis. 274 parents did not send the questionnaire back. Consequently, 1, 869 parent-adolescent dyads (Shantou: 1010; Ganzhou: 859) were finally included in the data analysis.

During the survey, adolescents in the grade 1 and grade 2 students in secondary school were invited to complete an anthropometric test for body weight and height, and were asked to fill out questionnaires inside a classroom with the assistance of an investigator. The adolescents were also asked to take home the "questionnaires for parents" for either their mother or father to fill out and report their own parenting behaviors, and to give the questionnaires back to the survey conductors. Souvenirs were given to the participants as compliments.

Prior to the conduct of the current study, 127 pairs (Ganzhou: 62 pairs, Shantou: 65 pairs) were invited to participate in a pilot study beforehand. During the pilot study, adolescents and their parents were required to complete the questionnaires twice with two weeks apart. The test-retest reliability of each item and internal consistency was determined by intraclass correlation coefficient and Cronbach's alpha respectively.

Signed informed consent was obtained from all participants (including adolescents and parents) prior to the survey. Formal approval was sought from the Chinese University of Hong Kong Research Ethics Committee.

## Main study measures

### Adolescent's age, gender and weight status

Adolescent gender and age were based on the adolescent's self-report. An adolescent's body weight and body height were measured by trained testers. Adolescents' age and gender specific body mass index Z scores (Z-BMI) were calculated based on the international growth standards for school-aged children and adolescents updated by the World Health Organization (WHO) (Butte, et al., 2007; De Onis, et al., 2007).

### Adolescents' self-reported dietary habits

Adolescents' dietary habits were measured by a five-point Likert-scale including 12 items. The adolescents were provided with responses ranging from "never," "rarely," "sometimes," "frequently," and "always" to indicate the frequency of their dietary behaviors during the past years. The sample questions were as follows: "I eat at least 3 servings of vegetables a day" and "I eat more during dinner if the food tastes good. " The total score of the adolescents' dietary habits was calculated as the sum score of each item. The validity and reliability of the scale were found to be acceptable (Sheu, 2003). The two weeks test-retest reliability of these items ranged from 0.70 to 0.79. The internal consistency for this scale was 0.71.

### Adolescents' self-reported physical activity level

All adolescents completed a validated physical activity rating questionnaire for children and youth (PARCY) to assess their average weekly physical activity over the last year. The PARCY is a 1-item activity rating modified from the Jackson Activity Coding (Baumgartner & Jackson, 1999; George, et al. , 1997) and the Godin-Shephard Activity Questionnaire modified for Adolescents (Aaron, et al. , 1993; Godin & Shephard, 1985). The scale is an 11 – point scale (0 – 10) ranging from no exercise at all (rating of 0) to doing vigorous exercise almost everyday (rating of 10). The design of the rating took into consideration activity frequency, duration, and intensity. The criterion validity and convergent validity of PARCY have been published in other sources (Hui, 2001; Hui, et al. , 2001; Kong, et al. , 2010). The two weeks test-retest reliability of the item was 0.83.

### Adolescents' self-reported pubertal status

Although it was suggested that obesity could be associated with pubertal timing (Kaplowitz, et al. , 2001; Tremblay & Frigon, 2005), pubertal status was not well controlled in many studies on adolescent obesity (Tsiros, et al. , 2008). In this study, a self-assessment questionnaire, which required the adolescents to report their pubic hair growth, breast development (for girls), and male genital development (for boys), was used to measure the children's pubertal status. The questionnaire enabled the reliable estimation of the sexual maturation status of Chinese children (Chan, et al. , 2008). The two weeks test-retest reliability of these two items in this study is 0.80 and 0.82, respectively. The internal consistency was 0.71.

### Adolescent-reported parenting style

Adolescents were required to report both their fathers' and mothers' parenting style via Authoritative Parenting Index (API), which was reported to have a factor structure consistent with a theoretical model of the construct and had good reliability (Jackson, et al. , 1998). There were nine items in the responsiveness subscale and seven items in the demandingness subscale. API was translated into Chinese and then back-translated into English to ensure the instrument's internal validity. The two weeks test-retest reliability of these items ranged from 0.70 to

0.85. The internal consistencies for the two subscales in fathers and mothers ranged from 0.70 tc 0.75, respectively. Scores for subscale of responsiveness and demandingness were calculated by summing the item scores. In addition, the data collected in the main survey was analyzed for construct validity. Confirmatory factor analysis usirg LISREL 8.51 software was conducted. The results of constructed validity test as well as the results of reliability test for this questionnaire showed that the factors loadings estimated based on the data of father and mothers were acceptable (ranged from 0.55 to 0.76 in fathers and ranged from 0.59 to 0.74 in mothers). The RMSEA, CFI and NNFI for the parenting style model also indicated acceptable fit. (based on fathers' data: RMSEA = 0.056, NNFI = 0.92, CFI = 0.93; based on mothers' data: RMSEA = 0.055, NNFI = 0.93, CFI = 0.94).

### Parent self-reported weight status

The BMIs of parents were recorded based on their self-reported heights and weights, as it is not feasible to measure parents' height and weight in the present study. The accuracy of the self-reported heights and weights of the adults collected from previous studies had been considered acceptable (Bolton-Smith, et al., 2000; Wada, et al., 2005).

### Self-reported parenting behaviors

An 17-item, five-point Likert-type scale, which was modified based on the questionnaires used in previous studies (Arredondo, et al., 2006; O'Connor, et al., 2010), was used to assess the parenting behaviors. The scale had the followings subscales: "diet and physical activity monitoring (MO)", "use food or sedentary behaviors as rewards (UR)", "pressure to eat (PE)", "restricting access to unhealthy food and sedentary behaviors (RA)", and "reinforcement (RF)" regarding adolescents' eating and PA. Five Likert-scale responses were provided for these questions (response options: never, rarely, sometimes, frequently, always or strongly disagree, disagree, neutral, agree, strongly agree). Another 1,000 data extracted randomly from the main survey was analyzed for constructed validity. Confirmatory factor analysis using LISREL 8.51 software was conducted. The description of the items as well as the results of construct validity test and reliability test were summarized in Table 3. 3 and Table 3. 6.

**Other information**

The background information supplied by the parents included parental education level, family income, and so on.

**Statistical Analysis**

Hierarchical multiple regressions were applied to examine moderator effects of parenting style on the association between parenting behaviors and adolescents' outcome ( dietary habits, physical activity and Z-BMI ). The procedures of regression followed the guideline for testing moderator effects ( Frazier, Tix, & Barron, 2004 ). Correlation coefficients among the variables were calculated and the variables found to be significantly associated with dependent variables were included in the models as covariates. All the variables were standardized before included in regression equation. Effects coding for categorical variables ( i. e. , codes of − 1 for male and 1 for female; code of − 1 for Ganzhou and 1 for Shantou ) was applied in the regression. Covariates were included in the first step of the regression equation, followed by independent variables, moderator variable, interaction between moderators and independent variables in subsequent steps. As multiple moderator effects were investigated in each model, all the moderator effects being considered were included in the same step in order to control Type I error. Interaction between covariates and other variables were tested in the final step. Recommended by Frazier et al. ( 2004 ), regression lines predicting the dependent variable ( adolescents' dietary habits, physical activity and Z-BMI ) were plotted, using the predicted values at low ( -1SD from the mean ) and high ( 1SD from the mean ) level of parenting behaviors in low and high parents' responsiveness ( or demanding ) groups. All the other variables in the model were fixed at 0. The details of the procedure was described elsewhere ( Frazier, et al. , 2004 ).

# 6.3 Results

2143 adolescents and 1869 their parents were included in this study. The age of adolescents recruited in this study ranged from 10 to 15. The descriptive statistics on adolescents' age, gender, BMI, dietary habits, physical activity, their parents' parenting behaviors and parenting style are summarized in Table 6. 1.

**Table 6. 1   General Characteristics of the Study Population**

| Adolescent sex | Percentage |
|---|---|
| Boy | 51. 4 |
| Girl | 48. 6 |
| Parent sex | |
| Male | 40. 4 |
| Female | 59. 6 |
| | Mean (SD) |
| Adolescent age, y | 12. 5 (0. 9) |
| Adolescents' BMI | 18. 6 (2. 8) |
| Adolescent dietary habits | 39. 3 (5. 3) |
| Adolescent physical activity | 5. 1 (2. 8) |
| Parent BMI | 22. 2 (3. 0) |
| Parenting behaviors | |
| Diet and physical activity monitoring (MO) | 19. 8 (4. 3) |
| Use food or sedentary behaviors as rewards (UR) | 5. 4 (1. 8) |
| Pressure to eat (PE) | 9. 8 (2. 1) |
| Restricting access to unhealthy food and sedentary behaviors (RA) | 15. 4 (2. 7) |
| Reinforcement (RF) | 7. 0 (2. 1) |
| Parenting style | |
| Responsiveness | 23. 9 (5. 6) |
| Demandingness | 17. 5 (5. 2) |

The results of regression show that, MO, RA, parents' responsiveness and demandingness were positively related to adolescents' dietary habits after adolescents' gender, age, parents' gender and location were adjusted (Table 2). The analysis also reveals that 10 % of variance of dietary habits were explained by the parenting behaviors and parenting styles. Additional 1% of the variance was explained by the interaction between parents' responsiveness and RA. Furthermore, the regression lines show that the positive relation between RA and adolescents' dietary habits was alleviated as parents' reponsiveness increased (Figure 6. 1A).

**Table 6.2  Prediction of Adolescents' Outcomes from Demographic Information, Parenting Behaviors and Parenting Style**

| | Dietary Habits | | | Physical Activity | | | Z – BMI | | |
|---|---|---|---|---|---|---|---|---|---|
| | B | 95% CI | $\Delta R^2$ | B | 95% CI | $\Delta R^2$ | B | 95% CI | $\Delta R^2$ |
| Step 1[a]: covariates | | | 0.03 | | | 0.09 | | | 0.10 |
| Adolescent's gender | 0.47** | 0.23, 0.71 | | −0.82** | −0.94, −0.69 | | −0.09 | −0.27, 0.08 | |
| Adolescent's Age | −0.57** | −0.82, −0.32 | | −0.20* | −0.33, −0.07 | | −0.29** | −0.49, −0.10 | |
| Parent's gender | 0.04 | −0.20, 0.29 | | 0.04 | −0.09, 0.17 | | −0.01 | −0.19, 0.17 | |
| Location | −0.67** | −1.17, −0.17 | | −0.90** | −1.17, −0.64 | | 0.04 | −0.33, 0.41 | |
| Adolescent's pubertal stage | N | N | | N | N | | 0.45** | 0.25, 0.65 | |
| Parent's BMI | N | N | | N | N | | 0.33** | 0.15, 0.50 | |
| Step 2: Predictors and moderators | | | 0.10 | | | 0.04 | | | 0.06 |
| MO | 0.64** | 0.24, 1.03 | | 0.27** | 0.08, 0.47 | | 0.18* | 0.04, 0.33 | |
| RF | −0.08 | −0.44, 0.28 | | −0.01 | −0.19, 0.16 | | 0.02 | −0.12, 0.15 | |
| UR | −0.14 | −0.52, 0.25 | | 0.00 | −0.06, 0.05 | | 0.25** | 0.11, 0.39 | |
| PE | −0.23 | −0.60, 0.15 | | N[b] | N[b] | | −0.50** | −0.64, −0.36 | |
| RA | 0.71** | 0.34, 1.09 | | 0.01 | −0.18, 0.19 | | 0.01 | −0.13, 0.15 | |

| | Dietary Habits | | | Physical Activity | | | Z − BMI | | |
|---|---|---|---|---|---|---|---|---|---|
| | B | 95% CI | $\Delta R^2$ | B | 95% CI | $\Delta R^2$ | B | 95% CI | $\Delta R^2$ |
| Responsiveness | 0.95** | 0.62, 1.28 | | 0.27** | 0.09, 0.44 | | 0.00 | -0.12, 0.12 | |
| Demandingness | 0.44* | 0.08, 0.79 | | 0.28*** | 0.12, 0.44 | | -0.09 | -0.22, 0.05 | |
| Step 3[a]: Predictors × moderators | | | 0.01 | | | 0.01 | | | 0.01 |
| RA × Responsiveness | -0.43* | -0.77, -0.08 | | N | N | | N | N | |
| MO × Demandingness | N | N | | 0.19* | 0.00, 0.39 | | 0.14* | 0.00, 0.28 | |
| Step 4[a]: Covariates × Other variables | | | 0.01 | | | 0.02 | | | 0.03 |
| Agender × RF | N | N | | 0.18* | 0.00, 0.37 | | N | N | |
| Age × Demandingness | N | N | | -0.18* | -0.35, -0.01 | | N | N | |
| Age × RA | N | N | | N | N | | -0.20** | -0.34, -0.05 | |
| Agender × PE | N | N | | N | N | | -0.17* | -0.31, -0.03 | |
| Agender × responsiveness | N | N | | N | N | | -0.12* | -0.24, 0.00 | |

Note: All the covariates, predictors and moderators were standardized before regression analysis. [a]: All the predictors × moderators, covariates × other variables were tested, but only the moderator effects with statistical significance were presented. [b]: PE (pressure to eat) was not included in the equation for physical activity prediction. N: The variable was not finally included in the model.

*: P <.05; **: P <.01

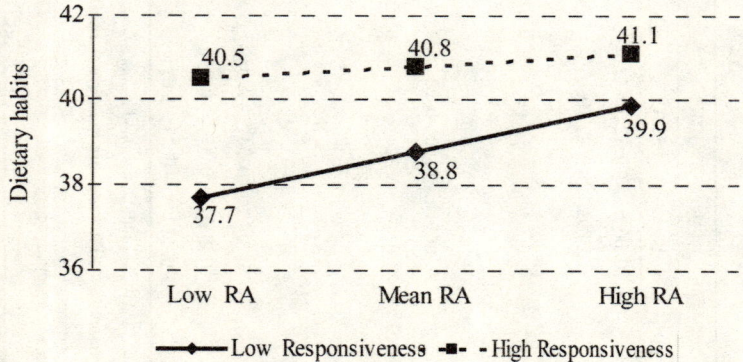

A: Relations between RA and adolescents' dietary habits as moderated by parents' responsiveness

The result shows that parents' responsiveness, demandingness and MO were found to be related to adolescents' physical activity. The interaction of parents' demandingness and MO was also found to be associated with adolescents' physical activity, although only 1% of the variance of adolescents' physical activity could be explained. It is also found that parents' high demandingness magnified the relationship between MO and adolescents' physical activity (Figure 6.1B).

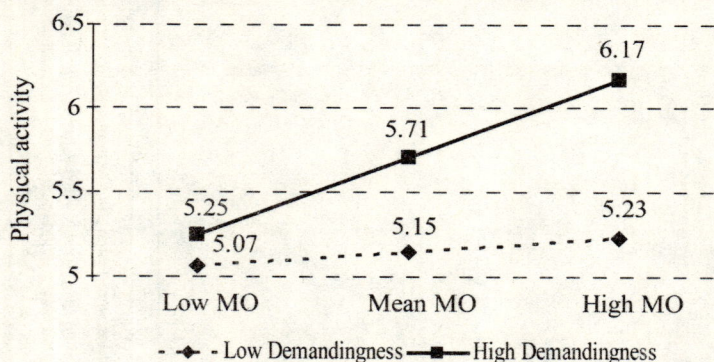

B. Relations between MO and adolescents' physical activity as moderated by parents' demandingness

MO, UR and PE were found to be significant predictors for adolescents' Z-

BMI. However, both parents' responsiveness and demandingness was not associated with adolescents' Z-BMI. The results revealed that the interaction of parents' demandingness and MO was significantly associated with adolescents' weight status, which explained 1% of the variance of adolescents' Z-BMI. In addition, parents' demandingness moderated the effects of MO on adolescents' weight status (Figure 6.1C).

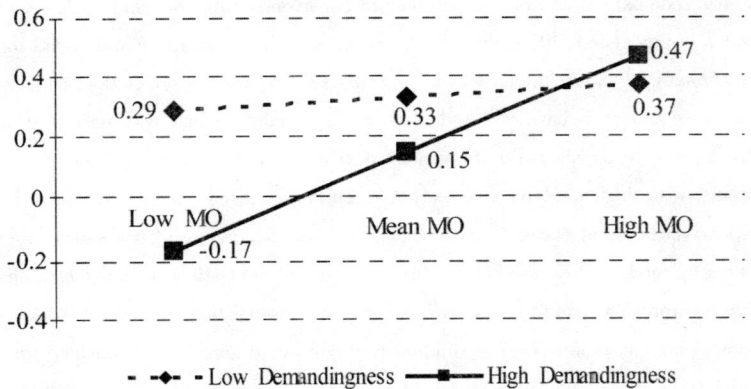

C. Relations between MO and adolescents' Z-BMI as moderated by parents' demandingness

**Figure 6.1  Regression lines for relations between parenting behaviors and adolescents' outcome as moderated by parenting style**

## 6.4   Discussion

To our knowledge, this is the first study to investigate the association among parenting behaviors, parenting style and adolescents' dietary habits, physical activity and weight status, based on the contextual model of parenting style recommended by Darling & Steinberg (1993). The findings confirmed that parenting style is a contextual variable that moderate the relationship between parenting behaviors and adolescents' outcome.

Parenting style was reported to play an important role in the children's diet.

For instance, a more demanding parenting style was found to be associated with lower consumption of sugar-sweetened beverages in adolescents (van der Horst, Kremers, et al., 2007). It was also reported that parents' use of appropriate disciplining styles was related to children's healthier eating (Arredondo, et al., 2006). Consistent with previous studies, current study also revealed that "food and physical activity monitoring", "restricting access to unhealthy food and youth's sedentary behaviors", parents' responsiveness and demandingness were positively associated adolescents' healthier eating. Furthermore, it was found that the strength of the relation between "restricting access to unhealthy food and youth's sedentary behaviors" and adolescents' dietary habits was increased by parents' low responsiveness. It suggested that, compared with the children of parents with higher responsiveness, the children raised by parents with low responsiveness were easier to have unhealthy diet if parents did not restrict their unhealthy food intake. Similarly, the results of present study also revealed that higher parents' demandingness may magnify the association between "food and physical activity monitoring" and adolescents' physical activity. It indicated that, compared with the adolescents raised by the parents with low demandingness, monitoring adolescents' physical activity could be more effective in the children of parents with higher demandingness.

Some parenting behaviors (such as food and physical activity monitoring) were associated with children's weight status (Faith, Berkowitz, et al., 2004). Maximizing (or minimizing) the effects of these parenting behaviors on children's weight status is very important in childhood obesity prevention. The data of this study suggests that the strength of the relationship between "food and physical activity monitoring" and adolescents' weight status could be increased by parents' demandingness, which may partly explain why the children of authoritative and authoritarian parents had lower ratios to be overweight (Rhee, et al., 2006; Wake, et al., 2007).

As it was suggested by contextual model of parenting style (Darling & Steinberg, 1993), parenting style may moderate the association between parenting behaviors and children's weight status in two paths. Firstly, parenting style may moderate the relationship by changing the nature of the parent-child interaction. It was found that good parent-child communication could be beneficial for parental monitoring ( Stattin & Kerr, 2000 ). Therefore, an authoritative parent may apply a more child-centered approach to monitor their children's food intake and physical activity as well as to prevent their children from unhealthy dietary habits and secentary behaviors. Secondly, good and respectful parent-child relationships may encourage adolescents to share their mental lives with their parents ( Stattin & Kerr, 2000 ). Darling and Steinberg ( 1993 ) also suggested that parenting style may influence adolescents' personality especially their openness to parenting practices, which in turn influence the effectiveness of parenting behaviors towards adolescents' dietary habits, physical activity and weight status.

In China, Confucianism dominated the content of traditional Chinese culture for centuries. In traditional Chinese families, there is a strong bond between parents and children, and parents could be the most influential people in the development of their child's lifestyle. Even today, although Chinese society has been greatly influenced by western culture, child rearing practices in China are still rooted in Confucianism ( Holroyd, 2003; P. Wu, et al. , 2002; Xu, et al. , 2005 ). Chinese parenting was often described as " authoritarian" , " restrictive" and " controlling" ( Lin & Fu, 1990; Steinberg, et al. , 1992 ). The studies based on Chinese parents showed that parenting style was associated with children's social and school performance ( Nelson, et al. , 2006 ) as well as child temperament ( Porter, et al. , 2005 ). The results of current study also indicated that parenting style may play an important role in the development of childhood obesity.

Several limitations need to be considered regarding the present study. First, although a relatively large sample was recruited in this study, the present research did not have a nationally representative design; therefore, the results may not be applied to all the Chinese. Other limitations may include the self-report nature of the data and the cross-sectional study design. Despite these limitations, the current study still successfully demonstrated that parenting style could moderate

313

the relation between adolescents' dietary habits, physical activity, weight status and parenting behaviors. This study highlights the indirect effects of parenting style on adolescents' weight status. The findings reported here suggest that the effects of parenting behaviors towards childhood obesity could be maximized when the moderating role of parenting style was considered.

# CHAPTER 7    GENERAL DISCUSSION AND CONCLUSION

During the past two decades, obesity among Chinese children became an increasing important public problem especially in urban areas of China (Luo & Hu, 2002). One of the important steps for childhood obesity prevention is to determine the factors associated with the development of children's weight problem. Studies indicated that parents may play important roles in the etiology and treatment of childhood obesity (Dietz & Robinson, 2005; Robinson, 1999). The aim of the present study was to determine the relationship among adolescents' weight status, parenting behaviors, parents' perception of their children's weight and parenting styles in China.

To obtain the objectives, our study was divided into two steps. For the first step, questionnaires to measure parents' perception of their children's weight, parenting behaviors, parenting styles for Chinese adolescents and their parents were validated. The present study successfully demonstrated that the content validity, construct validity, test retest reliability and internal consistency of the developed questionnaire were acceptable, and could be applied in adolescents and parents in sourthern China. For the second step, a cross-sectional survey was held to investigate the relationship among parenting behaviors, parents' perception of their children's weight, parenting styles, adolescents' dietary habits, physical activity and weight status in China. It was found that adolescents' weight status, dietary habits and physical activity were statistically significant but weakly associated with some parenting behaviors, including "pressure to eat", "resticting access to unhealthy food and sedentary behaviors", "diet and physical activity monitoring" and some other parenting behaviors. Moreover, parental perception of their

315

children's weight, which was found to be associated with parents' gender, adolescents' gender, and adolescents' perceptions of their own weights, could be related to some parenting behaviors related to the development of adolescent obesity. In addition, it was found that the adolescents' dietary habits, physical activity, and some parenting behaviors were associated with parenting style. However, we failed to find the direct association between parenting style and the adolescents' weight status. As several parent-related factors, including genetic factors, home environment and neighborhood built environment & safety and other factors, were not investigated in the present study, the model proposed may not comprehensively explain the relationship among the parent-related factors and adolescents' weight status. However, it is still believed that the findings in this study may help us better understand the association among parenting behaviors, parenting styles, parents' perceptions of their children's weight and adolescent obesity in China, which is very important for the etiology, development and treatment of Chinese adolescent obesity.

Given that the social environment and traditional culture in China is different from western countries, it was hypothesized that the influence of parents on their children's weight could be different from the results found in America and Europe. However, most of the results found in the present study were consistent with the findings reported in western countries. For example, although the prevalence of childhood obesity was still lower than developed countries ( Ji & Working Group on Obesity in China, 2005 ), Chinese parents did not show better ability in classifying their children's weights in this study. Moreover, in traditional Chinese culture, father and mother were arranged to play different parenting roles ( Berndt, et al. , 1993 ). However, the hypothesized gender differences in parenting behaviors were also not detected in the present study. The results maybe partly explained by the social change and influence of western culture in China during the past decades.

During the past a few years, parents involvement in the treatment of childhood obesity attracted many researchers' attention. Several scholars even promoted parents focused program, in which only parents were targeted in the intervention ( Golan & Weizman, 2001 ). The effectiveness of this kind of intervention were proved by some studies ( Golan & Crow, 2004b; McGarvey, et al. , 2004 ). However, the data of some other studies showed that parenting behaviors may only explain relatively low percentage of variance of children's food intake ( O'Connor, et al. , 2010 ) and physical activity ( Davison, Cutting, & Birch, 2003 ). The data of the current study confirmed that parenting behaviors, parenting style and parents' perception of their children's weight were associated with the development of adolescent obesity. However, the correlation is weak but statistically significant. Our data confirmed that parents involvement should be included in childhood obesity treatments ( Dietz & Robinson, 2005; Robinson, 1999 ). However, since parents related factors could only explain low percentage of adolescents' Z-BMI, dietary habits and physical activity, parents may only play an important supporting role rather than a leading role in the etiology, development and intervention of adolescent obesity.

Most current family studies of obesity concentrated on parental influence on their children's dietary habits, physical activity and weight status ( Anderssen & Wold, 1992; Heinberg, et al. , 2009; Moore, et al. , 1991; Savage, Fisher, & Birch, 2007; Wrotniak, et al. , 2004 ). In fact, the relationship between parents' and their children's could be bio-directional. For example, it was found that children may play an important role in helping their parents quit smoking ( Winickoff, et al. , 2006 ). Therefore, it is also possible for children to help their parents modify eating and physical activity behaviors, which could be applied in health promotion in adults. As a cross sectional study design was applied in the current study, cause and effect relationship can not be determined. Further studies were still needed to explore the role of parents in the development of childhood obesity as well as the influence of children on parents' behaviors.

In addition, adolescent-parent conflicts should be considered for the parents involvement in adolescent obesity treatment. A study based on Chinese adolescents and their parents suggested that adolescents want to have greater autonomy to make decision than their parents granted them ( Yau & Smetana, 1996 ). Three types of parent-child conflicts were found between the youth with eating disorders and their parents in mainland China, which include 1) intergenerational control and power struggle; 2) growing up versus remaining childlike, and 3) pursuit of personal goals or living up to parental expectations (J. L. C. Ma, 2008). As parents need to help their children modify their sedentary behaviors and unhealthy dietary habits, it is not surprising that the adolescent-parent conflicts may be increased, which could greatly influence the effectiveness of intervention. Therefore, adolescent-parent conflicts should be carefully dealt with and specific parenting skill training is recommended.

Although the results of the current study support that parent may play an important role in the development of adolescent obesity, some other factors, such as the influence of peer and school, should also be considered in the intervention of childhood obesity. Harmonious peer relationship not only provide important context for children's cognitive, psychological, and emotional development, but also influence children's physical activity, eating behaviors, and weight status (Salvy, et al. , 2008; Salvy, Howard, Read, & Mele, 2009; Storch, et al. , 2007). For instance, it was reported that children could do more vigorous physical activity in company of close friends (Salvy, et al. , 2008). Moreover, school may also influence children's weight status, through frequency and intensity of activity in physical education (The National Institute of Child Health Human Development Study of Early Child Care and Youth Development Network, 2003) as well as the food and soft drinks sold in schools (Committee on School Health, 2004). Therefore, the effects of intervention towards adolescent obesity would be maximized when all the relevant factors including parents, peer, school etc. are taken into account.

The limitations of this thesis may include the cross sectional study design, self-reported nature of survey data and non national representative sample. Therefore, in the present study, the cause and effect relationship can not be determined nor could the results be generalized in the Chinese all over the world. Longitudinal study design and objective instruments (eg. Using accelerators to measure PA, etc. ) were recommended in further studies.

In general, the data of the present study show that the questionnaires applied in the present study were reliable and valid. Parenting behaviors are weakly but significantly associated with the development of adolescent obesity. Misclassifications of children's weight status were prevalent among Chinese parents. Parental perceptions of their children's weights were associated with some parenting behaviors related to children's weight development. This study also highlights the indirect effects of parenting style on adolescents' weight status. The current study successfully demonstrated that parenting style could moderate the relation between adolescents' dietary habits, physical activity, weight status and parenting behaviors.

**图书在版编目（CIP）数据**

父母在青少年肥胖中的角色 / 温煦著.
—北京：中央编译出版社，2012.9
ISBN 978-7-5117-1466-4

Ⅰ.①父…

Ⅱ.①温…

Ⅲ.①家庭教育－关系－青少年－肥胖病－研究

Ⅳ.① G78 ② R589.2

中国版本图书馆 CIP 数据核字（2012）第 185649 号

**父母在青少年肥胖中的角色**

| | |
|---|---|
| 出 版 人 | 刘明清 |
| 出版统筹 | 薛晓源 |
| 责任编辑 | 王忠波　隋　丹 |
| 责任印制 | 尹　珺 |
| 出版发行 | 中央编译出版社 |
| 地　　址 | 北京西城区车公庄大街乙 5 号鸿儒大厦 B 座（100044） |
| 电　　话 | （010）52612345（总编室）　（010）52612339（编辑室） |
| | （010）66161011（团购部）　（010）52612332（网络销售） |
| | （010）66130345（发行部）　（010）66509618（读者服务部） |
| 网　　址 | www.cctpbook.com |
| 经　　销 | 全国新华书店 |
| 印　　刷 | 北京中印联印务有限公司 |
| 开　　本 | 880 毫米 × 1230 毫米　1/32 |
| 字　　数 | 217 千字 |
| 印　　张 | 10.5 |
| 版　　次 | 2012 年 9 月第 1 版第 1 次印刷 |
| 定　　价 | 58.00 元 |

本社常年法律顾问：北京市吴栾赵阎律师事务所律师　闫军　梁勤

凡有印装质量问题，本社负责调换，电话：（010）66509618